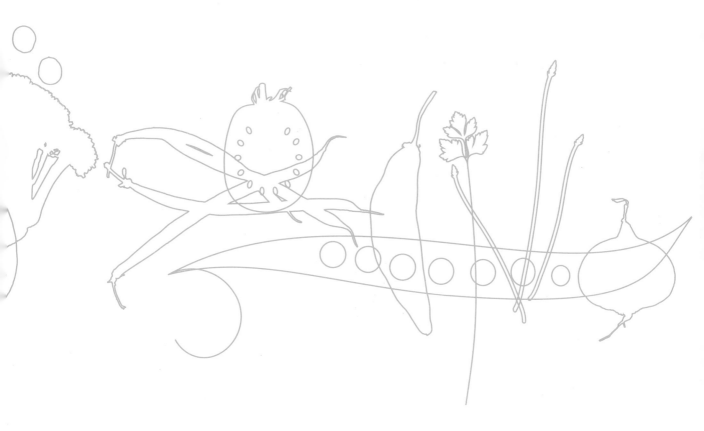

# PLENTY

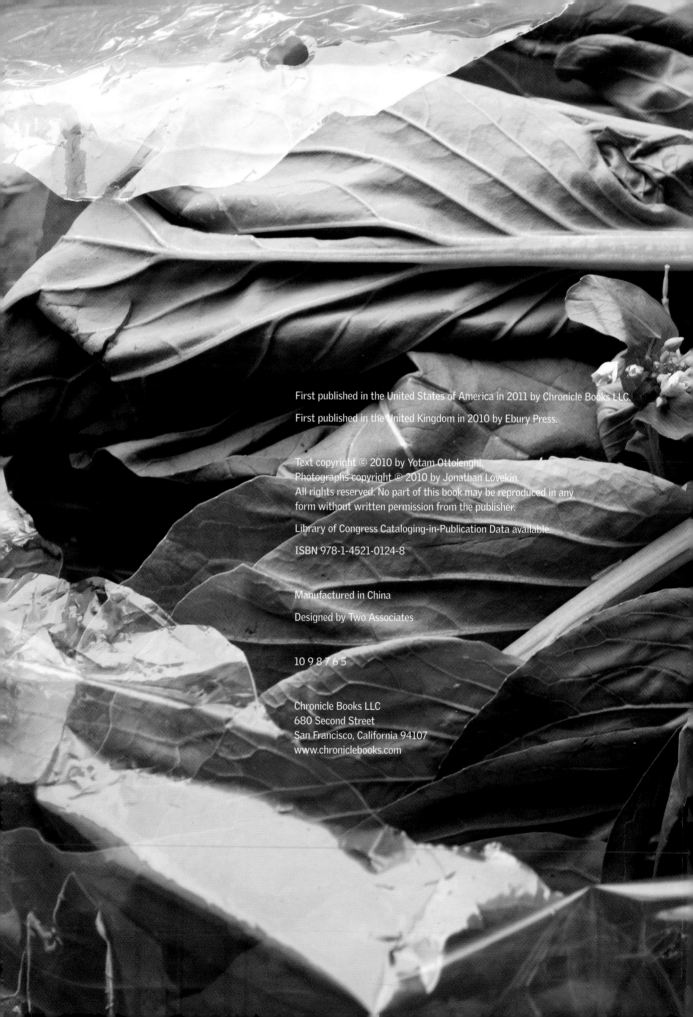

First published in the United States of America in 2011 by Chronicle Books LLC.

First published in the United Kingdom in 2010 by Ebury Press.

Text copyright © 2010 by Yotam Ottolenghi.
Photographs copyright © 2010 by Jonathan Lovekin.
All rights reserved. No part of this book may be reproduced in any
form without written permission from the publisher.

Library of Congress Cataloging-in-Publication Data available.

ISBN 978-1-4521-0124-8

Manufactured in China

Designed by Two Associates

10 9 8 7 6 5

Chronicle Books LLC
680 Second Street
San Francisco, California 94107
www.chroniclebooks.com

# PLENTY

## Vibrant Vegetable Recipes from London's Ottolenghi

## by YOTAM OTTOLENGHI

CHRONICLE BOOKS
San Francisco

# Contents

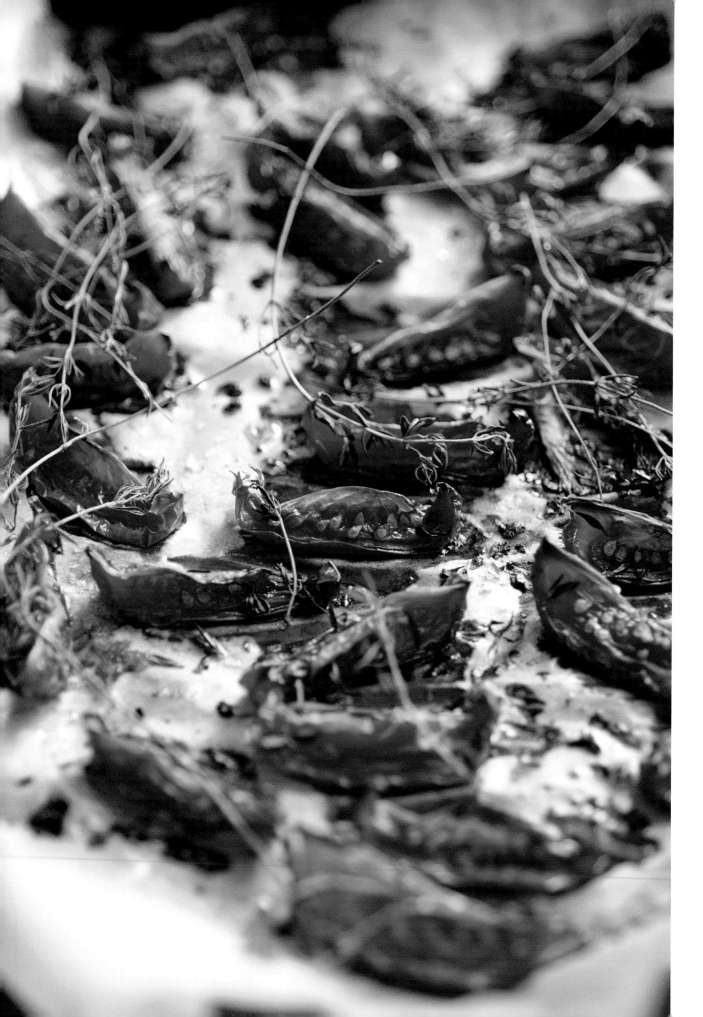

# Introduction

I'll start with something as simple and unassuming as rice. When I try to think of all the uses for this grain I immediately go dizzy with the countless possibilities – within and between cultures, pairing with other ingredients, all the types of rice available, the methods of cooking and when you serve it, the consistency, degree of processing, home cooking, commercial uses. I think of paella, wild rice salad and ho fan noodles. I visualize arancini with their golden breadcrumb crust, Iranian saffron rice with potatoes, Chinese fried rice, rice pudding. I recall plain steamed rice my mom used to prepare for me when I had a bad tummy, with only a little bit of butter stirred in at the end.

I can then move on to another cereal grain such as wheat and think of things we do with flour – dumplings, pastas, breads, pastries – or of less-processed examples like bulghur or whole wheat. My mind then wanders to the sphere of lentils, dried beans, green beans, peas. There are herbs, leaves, seeds, flowers, roots, bulbs, fruit and fungi – each part of a separate little universe, with a million varieties and variations within it.

What I am getting at is how lucky we are (although unfortunately not all of us) to be living and cooking in a world that offers such a spectrum of ingredients and so many culinary heritages to draw on. And this is what gets me excited – the multitude of ingredients cooked and processed by so many people in so many ways with so many different purposes.

## The New Vegetarian

Back in 2006, when I was first approached by the *Guardian* to write a vegetarian column in their *Weekend* magazine, I was slightly hesitant. After all, I wasn't a vegetarian. The issue wasn't close to my heart either and I had never given it much thought. Still, I understood the reasoning behind the *Guardian's* approach. Ottolenghi had become famous for what we did with vegetables and grains, for the freshness and originality of our salads, and it only made sense to ask me to share this with vegetarian readers.

It took me a while, though, to get to grips with my title, The New Vegetarian, and it made some *Guardian* readers extremely unhappy to learn that the new vegetarian wasn't a vegetarian at all. A couple of angry letters to the editor stick in my mind and an incident where I suggested serving a salad with some barbecued lamb chops. Unfortunately, my editor missed this too.

But with time the task has become more natural to me. Ottolenghi's vegetarian image was rightly based on the fact that both Sami Tamimi – the other creative force behind the company and co-author of *Ottolenghi: The Cookbook* – and I were brought up in Israel and Palestine and were exposed to the multitude of vegetables, pulses and grains that are celebrated in the region's different cuisines.

The food I had growing up was a huge mixture of diverse culinary cultures – European at home and Middle Eastern all around – with an abundance of easily sourced fresh ingredients. The greengrocer's where my mother does her shopping in the neighboring Arab village always reminds me of this. It sells a fantastically fresh abundance of local and seasonal fruit and veg, what I call real fruit and veg because they look real, taste real and are grown by real people – that is, Arab or Jewish farmers and not nameless farmers across the globe. It sells cucumbers, kohlrabis, figs, pomegranates, apricots, almonds and pistachios, as well as herbs from the area, local halva, olive oil and much more. Both my parents used this wealth daily to prepare real meals of real food, which is their food.

This multitude of ingredients and ways of making miracles with them have given me the perfect tools for making up dishes and turning them into recipes. This is also why vegetarian cooking didn't turn out to be a chore for me. I like meat and I like fish but I can easily cook without them. My grandmother's vinegar-marinated zucchini, or the ripe figs with sheep's cheese we used to down before dinner, are as substantial and as basic as any cut of meat I used to have.

## Vegetarianism

Still, I am not a vegetarian and this is important to mention. I refer to meat and fish in the introductions to the recipes as I occasionally have them in the back of my mind. But I don't miss these two elements. In this book I offer dozens of solid dishes, all balanced and nurturing, that just happen to include neither fish nor meat.

Why vegetarianism then? What is the reason behind not having meat or fish? Why would people be interested in this vegetarian collection?

First, this is an assembly of my work in the *Guardian* over the past four years. I have often been asked by readers, who've become fed up with collecting little bits of torn paper, to assemble it all together in one volume. Most of these bits of paper are now here for them, plus plenty more new recipes I haven't published before.

But more to the point, people have very different motivations for wanting to cook vegetarian recipes. Some choose unequivocally to exclude meat from their diet. Many do this for moral or other personal reasons, which I both understand and respect. These people may find allusions to non-vegetarian ingredients disturbing. Some may not like my extensive use of eggs and dairy products. Many would probably be put off by my advocating the use of Parmesan and other continental cheeses that almost always include animal rennet in their production. My answer to all these objections is that I can only be myself and cook what I like to eat. I believe that most seasoned vegetarians would know which elements in the book to adopt and which to disregard, which suit their type of vegetarianism and which don't.

A second group of people, which is increasingly growing in number, are pragmatic vegetarians, those who have excluded meat or fish from their diet to some degree, but are not completely put off by the notion. This group would include people who are concerned with the health implications of eating meat. It also consists of people who would like to eliminate or reduce their consumption of meat and fish due to the environmental implications. They are put off by what mass-scale farming does to the land and the sea, how growing numbers of cattle herds contribute to the growth in greenhouse gases and the warming up of the planet. Many long for a time when meat was precious, a reason for celebration rather than a cheap commodity, a time when farm animals were highly regarded and their slaughter more sensible.

Recent campaigns for the reduced consumption of meat emphasize how wasteful it is to gain our calories from meat rather than from vegetables, pulses or grains. This argument and the general sense of over-indulgence over the last few decades have convinced many to include less meat in their diet, to make it special and valuable again.

This, along with increased availability of old and new vegetables and the knowledge of how to grow them or source them ethically, is the most important force behind the heightened interest in vegetarian food.

## The Book

I divided this book into chapters in quite an unsystematic way. More than anything, it reveals the way I think and work when writing a recipe. At the center of every dish, at the beginning of the thought process, is an ingredient, one ingredient – not just any ingredient but one of my favorite ingredients. I tend to set off with this central element and then try to elaborate on it, enhance it, bring it out in a new way, while still keeping it in the center, at the heart of the final dish.

So the chapters reflect this bias. They focus on some ingredients and neglect others, and they hold them together in clusters that make sense to me. Some components are so central to my cooking – like eggplant, of course – that I dedicate a special chapter to them alone. Then there are botanical categories, like brassicas, that although a little scientific actually make sense to me; they bring together vegetables that I naturally associate with each other, earthy yet fresh. Other headings stem from other private associations and the way I shape my menus.

Many of the recipes that were published before, mainly in the *Guardian*, have had some changes made to them, some more radical than others. I can't always recount why these changes were made. My style of cooking and writing has changed over the years and things that seemed to make sense then (potato in an artichoke gratin, for example) don't make sense now. But more generally, every time you approach a dish, at least when I do, it feels slightly different. It seems to be asking for a little alteration, for the addition of this or the removal of that. I try to stay attentive to this. I guess this is what makes real food.

## Yotam Ottolenghi

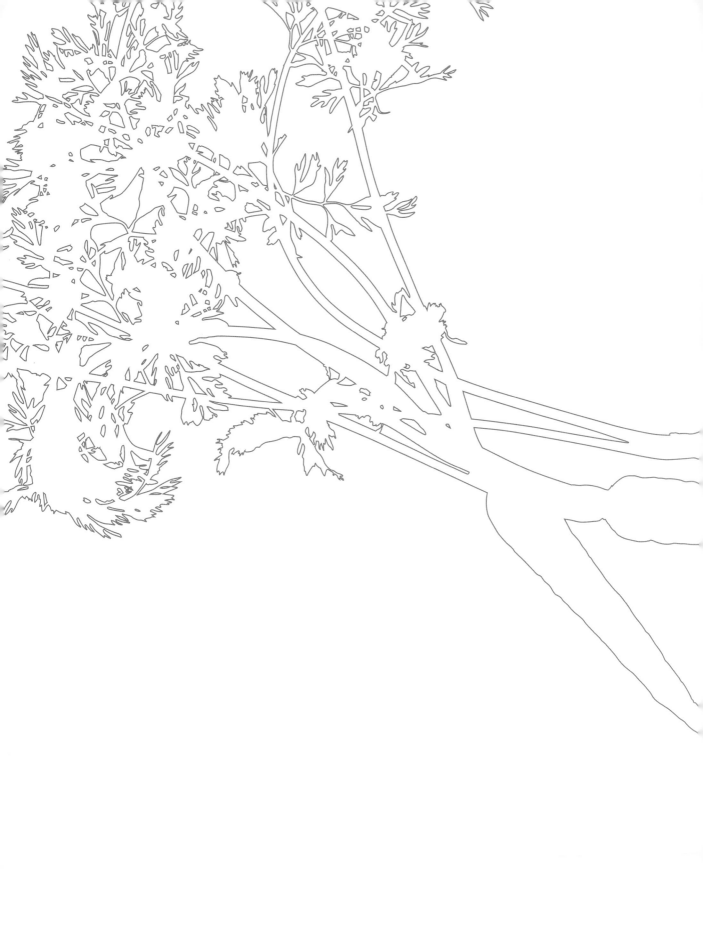

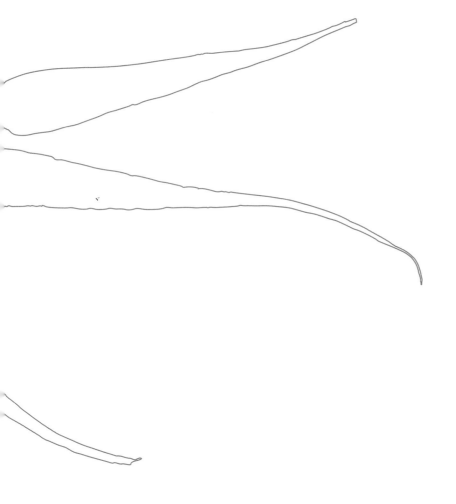

Roots

# Poached baby vegetables with caper mayonnaise

Poaching is popular again, and rightly so. Vegetables cooked this way don't need to be insipid or dull; if not overcooked, they can show off their natural attributes and taste fresh and light in a way that you never get when roasting or frying.

When making this recipe, choose beautiful seasonal vegetables that are clearly fresh and flavorful. Baby turnips or corn will work too, and you can also add fresh fava beans, peas and green beans. Just remember to give your vegetables minimum treatment – don't chop them up much and don't cook them for very long. Serve the vegetables warm or cold.

Serves 4

Mayonnaise
½ garlic clove, crushed
1 egg yolk
1½ tsp white wine vinegar
½ tsp Dijon mustard
½ tsp salt
grated zest and juice of ½ lemon
⅓ cup vegetable oil
2 tbsp capers, drained well and finely
    chopped

1 bunch baby carrots, peeled
4 baby fennel
12 spears fine asparagus
8 baby zucchini
10 baby leeks
2 tbsp chopped dill to serve

Poaching liquor
2½ cups white wine
1 cup olive oil
⅔ cup lemon juice
2 bay leaves
½ onion
2 celery stalks
1 tsp salt

To make the mayonnaise. Place the garlic, egg yolk, vinegar, mustard, salt and lemon juice in the bowl of a food processor. Start blending and then very slowly dribble in the oil until you get a thick mayonnaise. Fold in the capers and lemon zest and set aside.

Wash the vegetables but don't trim them too much so you are left with some of the stalk or leaves. Cut the vegetables lengthways into halves or quarters, depending on their size, trying to get similarly sized pieces. Very thin vegetables, like asparagus, don't need to be cut.

To make the poaching liquor. Place the wine in a wide pan and boil for 2 to 3 minutes. Add all the other poaching liquor ingredients and bring to a simmer. Start the poaching by adding the carrots and fennel to the pot. After 3 minutes add the asparagus, zucchini and leeks and poach for a further 3 to 4 minutes. At this point the vegetables should be cooked but still crunchy.

Using tongs lift the vegetables from the poaching liquor and onto deep plates. Spoon some liquor around the vegetables if you like. Before serving, top each portion with a dollop of mayonnaise and sprinkle with dill. You can keep the remaining poaching liquor in the fridge to use again.

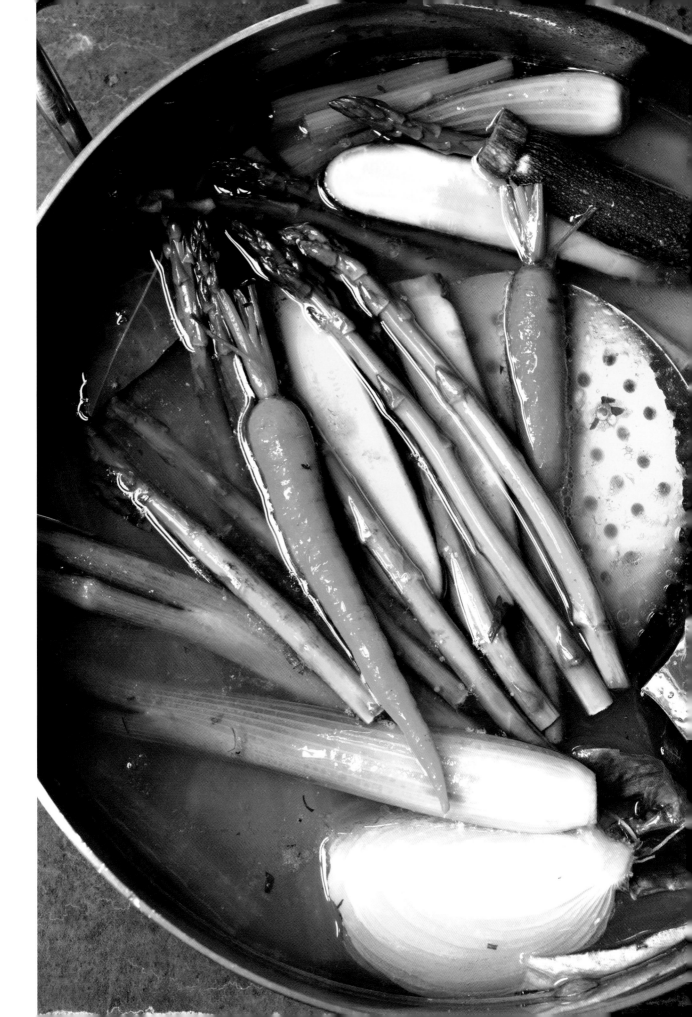

# Spicy Moroccan carrot salad

There are countless variations on this gutsy salad, all incorporating sweet spices, fresh herbs and some sort of lemony kick. My version is intense and will go well as one component in a feast of Middle Eastern salads, or just to accompany fried fish. You can serve it warm, as well as cold, with Freekeh Pilaf (page 241) for instance.

Serves 4

2 lbs carrots
⅓ cup olive oil, plus extra to finish
1 medium onion, finely chopped
1 tsp sugar
3 garlic cloves, crushed
2 medium green chiles, finely chopped
1 green onion, finely chopped
⅛ tsp ground cloves
¼ tsp ground ginger
½ tsp ground coriander
¾ tsp ground cinnamon
1 tsp sweet paprika
1 tsp ground cumin
1 tbsp white wine vinegar
1 tbsp chopped preserved lemon
salt
2½ cups cilantro leaves, chopped,
    plus extra to garnish
½ cup Greek yogurt, chilled

Peel the carrots and cut them, depending on their size, into cylinders or semicircles ½ inch thick; all the pieces should end up roughly the same size. Place in a large saucepan and cover with salted water. Bring to the boil, then turn down the heat and simmer for about 10 minutes or until tender but still crunchy. Drain in a colander and leave to dry out.

Heat the oil in a large pan and sauté the onion for 12 minutes on a medium heat until soft and slightly brown. Add the cooked carrots to the onion, followed by all the remaining ingredients, apart from the cilantro and yogurt. Remove from the heat. Season liberally with salt, stir well and leave to cool.

Before serving, stir in the cilantro, taste and adjust the seasoning if necessary. Serve in individual bowls with a dollop of yogurt, a drizzle of oil and garnished with the extra cilantro.

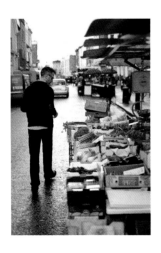
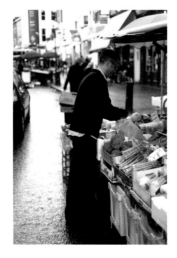
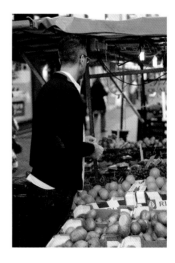

# Beet, orange and black olive salad

The mild sweetness of beets offers an ideal background for the intensity of sharp orange and salty olive, creating an unusual yet delicious salad. Use Greek black olives of the dry, wrinkled variety. Having matured longer on the tree, they are saltier and more robust in flavor. If you wish to keep the salad more mild and fresh it also tastes great without the olives. Serve with Steamed Rice with Herbs (page 235) to create a light and healthful meal.

Serves 2 generously
5 small or 2 large beets
2 oranges
1 Treviso (red chicory)
½ small red onion, thinly sliced
3 tbsp chopped parsley
5 tbsp black olives, pitted and halved
3 tbsp grapeseed oil
1 tsp orange flower water
1½ tbsp red wine vinegar
salt and black pepper

Place the beets in a pot, cover with cold water and bring to the boil. Cook for 1 to 2 hours, or until tender – when you stick a small knife into each beet it should go in smoothly. Leave the beets to cool down in the water. Once cool, take them out and peel. Cut in half, then cut each half into wedges that are 1 inch thick at their base. Place the beets in a mixing bowl.

Take the oranges and use a small sharp knife to trim off their tops and bases. Now cut down the sides of the oranges, following their natural curves, to remove the skin and white pith. Over a small bowl remove the segments from the oranges by slicing between the membranes. Transfer the segments and juice to the bowl with the beets; discard the membrane.

Cut the Treviso vertically into 1-inch-thick slices. Break them up into separate leaves and add to the salad.

Finally, add the remaining ingredients and toss everything together gently. Taste and adjust the seasoning, then serve.

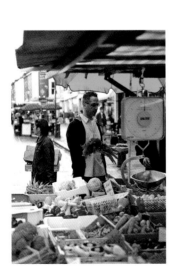
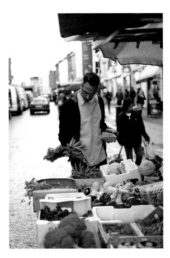
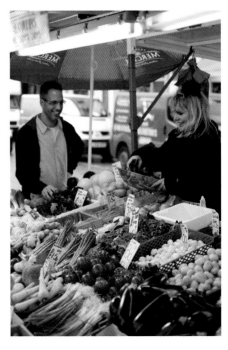

# Roasted parsnips and sweet potatoes with caper vinaigrette

Treat this recipe as a blueprint for an infinite number of roast vegetable dishes. The point here is to lighten up long-cooked veggies with something crisp and fresh. You can use any of your favorite vegetables – rutabaga, potato, carrot, salsify, beet, cauliflower – and many other refreshing combinations at the end: chopped herbs such as basil or mint, grated lemon zest, harissa paste, crushed garlic or a mellow vinegar.

Serves 4

4 parsnips (1½ lbs total)
4 medium red onions
⅔ cup olive oil
4 thyme sprigs
2 rosemary sprigs
1 head garlic, halved horizontally
salt and black pepper
2 medium sweet potatoes (1¼ lbs total)
30 cherry tomatoes, halved
2 tbsp lemon juice
4 tbsp small capers (roughly chopped if large)
½ tbsp maple syrup
½ tsp Dijon mustard
1 tbsp toasted sesame seeds (optional)

Preheat the oven to 375°F. Peel the parsnips and cut into two or three segments, depending on their lengths. Then cut each piece lengthways into two or four. You want pieces roughly 2 inches long and ½-inch wide. Peel the onions and cut each into six wedges.

Place the parsnips and onions in a large mixing bowl and add ½ cup of the olive oil, the thyme, rosemary, garlic, 1 teaspoon salt and some pepper. Mix well and spread out in a large roasting pan. Roast for 20 minutes.

While the parsnips are cooking, trim both ends of the sweet potatoes. Cut them (with their skins) widthways in half, then each half into six wedges. Add the potatoes to the pan with the parsnips and onion and stir well. Return to the oven to roast for a further 40 to 50 minutes.

When all the vegetables are cooked through and have taken on a golden color, stir in the halved tomatoes. Roast for 10 minutes more. Meanwhile, whisk together the lemon juice, capers, maple syrup, mustard, remaining 2 tablespoons oil and ½ teaspoon salt.

Pour the dressing over the roasted vegetables as soon as you take them out of the oven. Stir well, then taste and adjust the seasoning. Scatter the sesame seeds over the vegetables if using and serve at the table in the roasting pan.

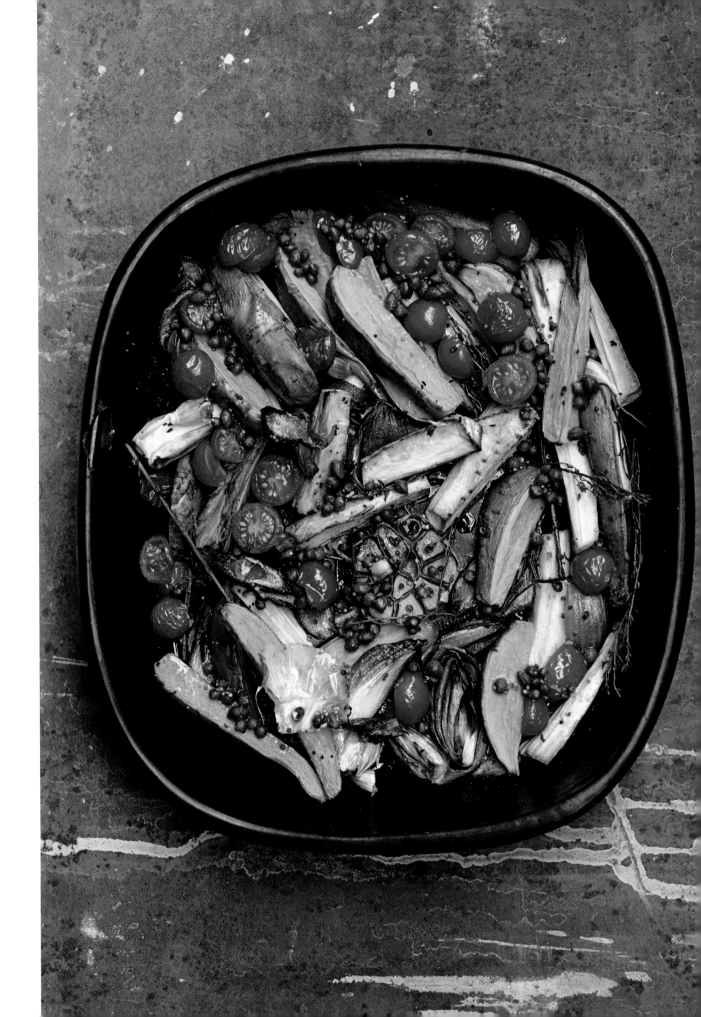

# Two-potato vindaloo

Here's a great recipe you can make heaps of and keep for a few days. It only gets better! As always, thick cool yogurt will make an excellent condiment.

Serves 4

8 cardamom pods
1 tbsp cumin seeds
1 tbsp coriander seeds
½ tsp cloves
¼ tsp ground turmeric
1 tsp sweet paprika
1 tsp ground cinnamon
2 tbsp vegetable oil
12 shallots (about 10 oz in total), chopped
½ tsp brown mustard seeds
½ tsp fenugreek seeds
25 curry leaves
2 tbsp chopped fresh ginger
1 fresh red chile, finely chopped
3 ripe tomatoes, peeled and roughly chopped
¼ cup cider vinegar
1¾ cups water
1 tbsp sugar
salt
2½ cups peeled waxy potatoes, cut into 1-inch dice
2 small red bell peppers, cut into 1-inch dice
2½ cups peeled sweet potatoes, cut into 1-inch dice
mint or cilantro leaves to serve

Dry-roast the cardamom pods and cumin and coriander seeds in a small frying pan over medium heat until they begin to pop. Transfer to a mortar and pestle and add the cloves. Work to a fine powder, removing and discarding the cardamom pods once the seeds are released. Add the turmeric, paprika and cinnamon and set aside.

Heat up the oil in a large heavy-based pot. Add the shallots with the mustard and fenugreek seeds, and sauté on a medium–low heat for 8 minutes, or until the shallots brown. Stir in the spice mix, curry leaves, ginger and chile and cook for a further 3 minutes. Next, add the tomatoes, vinegar, water, sugar and some salt. Bring to the boil, then leave to simmer, covered, for 20 minutes.

Add the potatoes and bell peppers and simmer for another 20 minutes. For the last stage, add the sweet potatoes. Make sure all the vegetables are just immersed in the sauce (add more water if needed) and continue cooking, covered, for about 40 minutes, or until the potatoes are tender.

Remove the lid and leave to bubble away for about 10 minutes to reduce and thicken the sauce. Serve hot, with plain rice and garnished with herbs.

# Beet, yogurt and preserved lemon relish

Some wonderful beets are available in the summer months: small, firm bulbs, sold with the stalks and the leaves. Don't throw out the leaves. Use them for salads, or sauté with a little olive oil, garlic and caraway seeds and serve warm with a dollop of crème fraîche. If you manage to get young beets you may want to roast them in the oven, covered in foil, rather than boil them as described below. They are more flavorful this way.

The preserved lemon relish can be used in loads of other contexts. Try mixing with cooked potato to create a salad or serving alongside oily fish.

Serves 4
2 lbs large beets
4 heaped tbsp chopped dill
1 small red onion, very thinly sliced
⅔ cup Greek yogurt

Relish
2 yellow bell peppers
3 tbsp olive oil
1½ tsp coriander seeds
one 14-oz can chopped plum tomatoes
    (with their juices)
2 garlic cloves, crushed
1 tsp sugar
salt and black pepper
3 tbsp chopped preserved lemon
2 tbsp each chopped parsley and
    cilantro

Start by cooking the beets whole in plenty of boiling water for 1 to 2 hours, or until they are tender; check by piercing them with a knife. Allow them to cool down completely before you peel them and cut into wedges.

To make the relish. Preheat the grill to high. Use a small knife to cut around the stems of the peppers; carefully pull out the stems with the seeds and discard. Place the peppers on a grill pan lined with foil and grill for up to 30 minutes, or until they are cooked inside and black on the outside, turning them over once during the cooking. Fold the edges of the foil over the peppers to enclose them completely, then leave to cool down. Peel them and cut into strips.

Pour the olive oil into a medium saucepan, heat up and fry the coriander seeds for 30 seconds. Add the tomatoes, garlic, sugar and some salt and pepper and simmer for 15 minutes. Add the preserved lemon and continue simmering for 10 minutes. Remove from the heat and stir in the herbs and yellow pepper strips. Allow to cool down completely.

When you are ready to finish the salad, transfer the cool beet wedges to a mixing bowl and add the relish, dill, red onion and some salt and pepper. Stir well, then taste for seasoning. Just before you serve, add the yogurt and swirl it through gently. Don't stir too much, so you get a white and red marbled effect rather than uniform pink.

# Royal potato salad

Jersey Royal potatoes are at their peak in spring and early summer, which is just as well since they make a stunning picnic salad. This one is a poshed-up version of the ordinary spud salad and it's just as satisfying.

Serves 4–6

15 quail's eggs

1 cup petite peas (frozen)

1¾ lbs new potatoes, such as Jersey Royals, washed but not scrubbed

1 cup basil leaves

½ cup parsley leaves, plus a little extra chopped to garnish

⅓ cup pine nuts

½ cup grated Parmesan (2 oz)

2 garlic cloves, crushed

1 cup olive oil

½ tsp white wine vinegar

bunch of sorrel (or mint) leaves, finely shredded

salt and black pepper

Place the quail's eggs in a saucepan, cover with cold water and bring to the boil. Simmer for between 30 seconds (soft-boiled) and 2 minutes (hard-boiled), depending on how you like them cooked. Refresh in cold water, then peel.

Blanch the peas in boiling water for 30 seconds, then drain and refresh. Set aside.

In a separate pan of boiling water, cook the potatoes for 15 to 20 minutes, or until they are soft but not falling apart.

While the potatoes are cooking place the basil, parsley, pine nuts, Parmesan and garlic in a food processor and blitz to a paste. Add the oil and pulse until you get a runny pesto. Pour into a large bowl.

Drain the potatoes, then cut in two as soon as you can handle them (they will absorb more flavor when hot). Add to the bowl and toss with the pesto, vinegar, sorrel and peas. Mix well, even crushing the potatoes slightly, so all the flavors mix. Taste and adjust the seasoning; be generous with pepper.

Cut the eggs in half and gently fold into the salad. Garnish with chopped parsley.

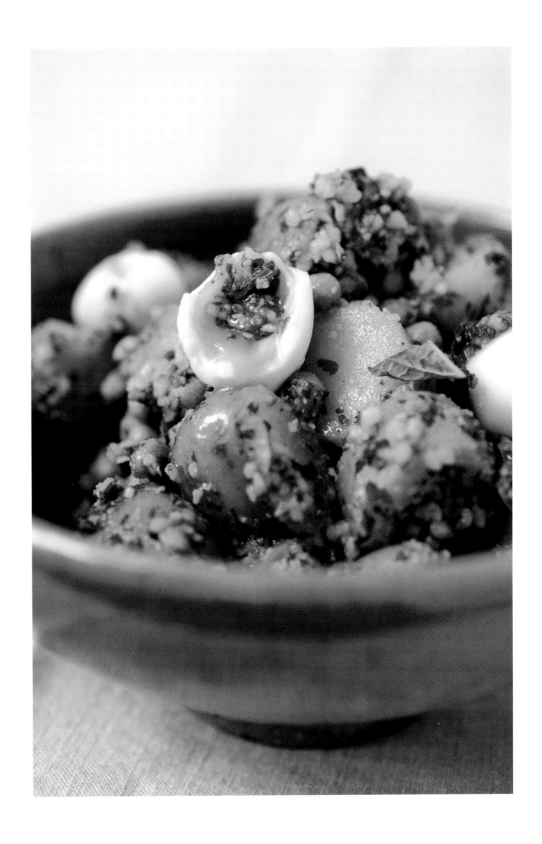

# Surprise tatin

Filling a tart with potatoes is a real treat for potato lovers. Serve it with a green salad and you don't need much else. You can use commercial sun-dried tomatoes in oil to save yourself making the oven-dried tomatoes.

Serves 4

1½ cups cherry tomatoes

2 tbsp olive oil, plus extra for drizzling over the tomatoes and for the pan

salt and black pepper

1 lb new potatoes (skins on)

1 large onion, thinly sliced

3 tbsp sugar

2 tsp butter

3 oregano sprigs

5 oz aged goat cheese, sliced

1 puff pastry sheet, rolled thinly

Preheat the oven to 275°F. Halve the tomatoes and place them skin-side down on a baking sheet. Drizzle over some olive oil and sprinkle with salt and pepper. Place in the oven to dry for 45 minutes.

Meanwhile, cook the potatoes in boiling salted water for 25 minutes. Drain and let cool. Trim off a bit of the top and bottom of each potato, then cut into 1-inch-thick discs.

Sauté the onion with the oil and some salt for about 10 minutes, or until golden brown.

Once you've prepared all the vegetables, brush a 9-inch cake pan with oil and line the bottom with a circle of parchment paper. In a small pan cook the sugar and butter on a high heat, stirring constantly with a wooden spoon, to get a semi-dark caramel. Pour the caramel carefully into the cake pan and tilt it to spread the caramel evenly over the bottom. Pick the oregano leaves, tear and scatter on the caramel.

Lay the potato slices close together, cut-side down, on the bottom of the pan. Gently press onion and tomatoes into the gaps and sprinkle generously with salt and pepper. Spread the slices of goat cheese evenly over the potatoes. Cut a puff pastry disc that is 1 inch larger in diameter than the pan. Lay the pastry lid over the tart filling and gently tuck the edges down around the potatoes inside the pan. (At this stage you can chill the tart for up to 24 hours.)

Preheat the oven to 400°F. Bake the tart for 25 minutes, then reduce the temperature to 350°F and continue baking for 15 minutes, or until the pastry is thoroughly cooked. Remove from the oven and let settle for 2 minutes only. Hold an inverted plate firmly on top of the pan and carefully but briskly turn them over together, then lift off the pan. Serve the tart hot or warm.

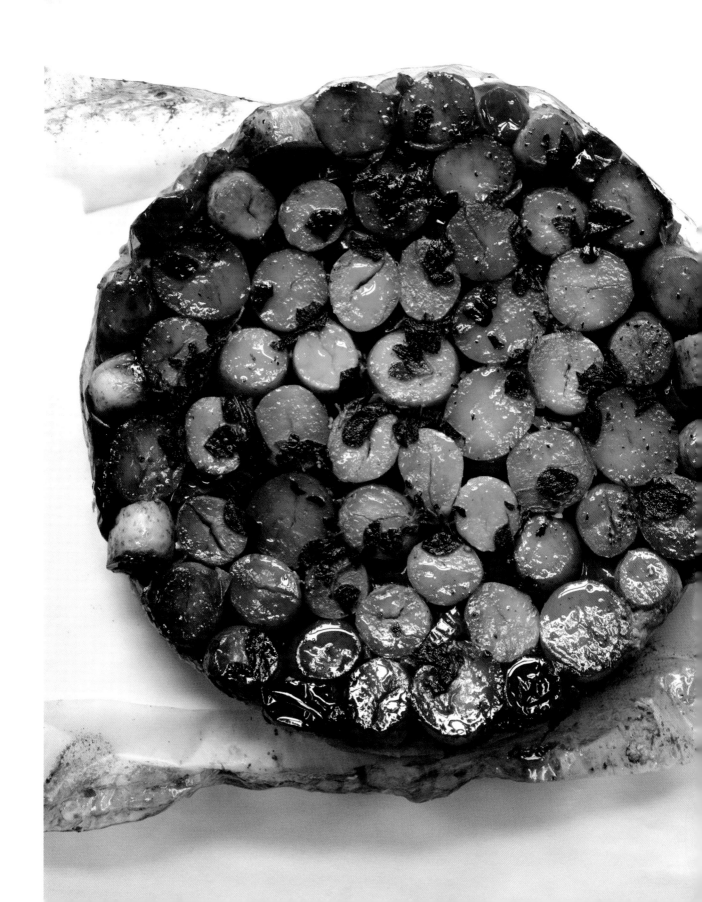

# Jerusalem artichokes with Manouri and basil oil

Here's a complex salad that makes a whole satisfying meal on its own. In its center there is Manouri, a rich Greek sheep's cheese that I use often. If you can't get it, use halloumi or another softish, young sheep's cheese.

Serves 4
1 lb Jerusalem artichokes
juice of 2 small lemons
4 thyme sprigs
1 tbsp olive oil
salt and black pepper

Basil oil
2 cups basil (leaves and stalks)
½ cup flat-leaf parsley (leaves and
    stalks)
1 garlic clove, peeled
salt
⅔ cup olive oil

½ cup olive oil
2¾ cups cherry tomatoes
salt
14 oz Manouri cheese (or halloumi), cut
    into ½-inch-thick slices
1 Treviso or Belgian endive (red or white
    chicory), separated into leaves

Preheat the oven to 425°F. Start with the artichokes. Squeeze the juice of 1 lemon into a medium bowl and add about 2¼ cups of water. Peel the artichokes with a vegetable peeler, slice them lengthways ⅜-inch thick and throw immediately into the acidulated water to prevent them from turning brown.

Lift the artichokes from the water into an ovenproof dish. Add the thyme, the juice of the second lemon, 3 tablespoons water, 1 tablespoon olive oil and some salt and pepper. Mix everything together, then spread out the artichoke slices. Cover the dish with foil and put it into the oven to roast for 40 to 45 minutes, or until the artichokes are tender. Take out of the oven and keep somewhere warm.

To make the basil oil. Put the basil, parsley, garlic and a pinch of salt in a food processor bowl and start the machine. Add the oil in a slow trickle. When it is all incorporated you will have a runny paste.

Place a large frying pan on high heat and let it heat up well. Add 1 tablespoon of the oil and the tomatoes and char them quickly, shaking the pan to get even coloring. After 3 to 4 minutes the tomatoes should be lightly blackened but retain their shape. Sprinkle with salt, remove from the pan and add them to the cooked artichokes.

When you are ready to serve, wipe clean your frying pan and pour in enough olive oil to come 2 inches up the sides. Set on a medium heat and, once hot, fry the cheese slices for about 2 minutes on each side, or until they turn a good brown color. Transfer to paper towels.

Arrange some endive leaves on serving dishes. Build up the salad on top with warm cheese, Jerusalem artichokes, cherry tomatoes and more leaves. Finish with a drizzle of basil oil and serve at once.

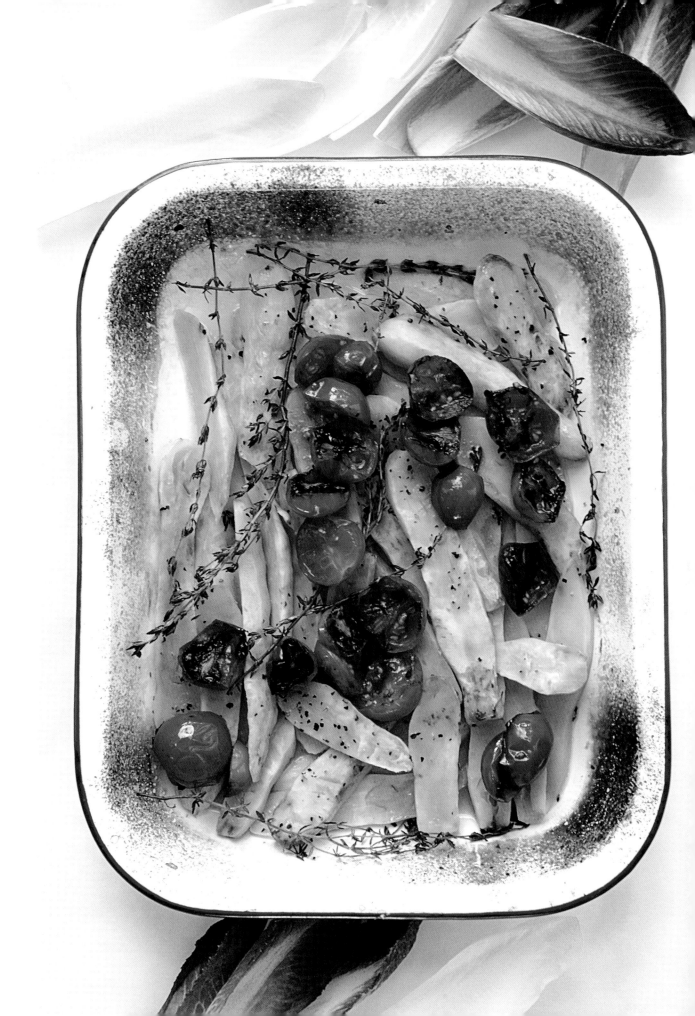

# Sweet potato wedges with lemongrass crème fraîche

My right-hand person with this book was Claudine Boulstridge. Claudine tried most of the recipes diligently and came back with criticisms, insights and general common-sensical observations. Despite her gracious nature I could always rely on her to tell me if something I'd come up with was utter rubbish. To top it all, she is also very creative. This is one of her recipes and it's wonderful.

Serves 4
3 medium sweet potatoes (about 2 lbs in total)
4 tbsp olive oil
1½ tsp ground coriander
¾ tsp fine sea salt
1 fresh red chile, finely diced
1 cup cilantro, leaves picked

Dipping sauce
½ lemongrass stalk
¾ cup crème fraîche
grated zest and juice of 2 limes
1 inch fresh ginger, peeled and grated
½ tsp fine sea salt

Preheat the oven to 400°F. Wash the sweet potatoes but don't peel them. Cut each lengthways in half. Cut again lengthways into quarters and then once more in the same way, so you are left in the end with eight long wedges.

Place them in a roasting pan that has been lined with parchment paper and brushed lightly with some of the olive oil. Brush the wedges with the remaining oil and sprinkle with a mixture of the ground coriander and salt. Roast for about 25 minutes, or until the sweet potato is tender and golden brown. Remove from the oven and allow to cool down a little. (The wedges can be eaten warm or at room temperature.)

To make the dipping sauce. Very finely chop the lemongrass or grind finely in a spice grinder. Whisk with all of the other ingredients for the dipping sauce and set aside.

When ready to serve, place the wedges on a large, flat serving dish. Sprinkle with the diced chile and cilantro leaves, and serve with the sauce on the side.

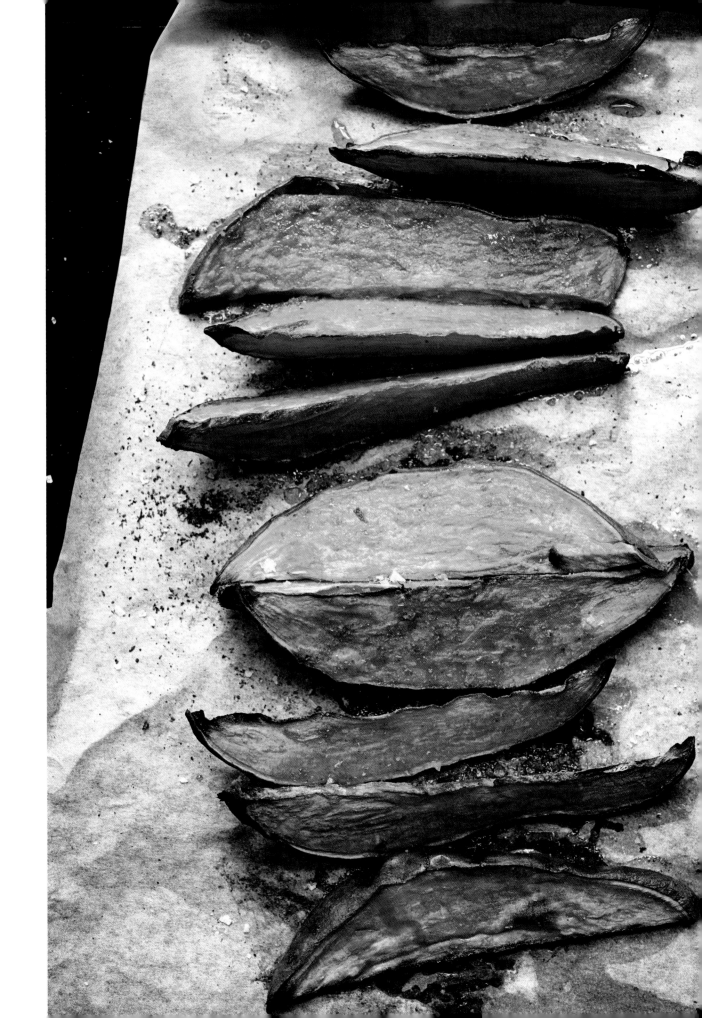

# Parsnip dumplings in broth

Ossi Burger, a dear friend who is famous for her lavish meals, always comes up with ingenious solutions for the one and only vegetarian in the bunch, her daughter Noa. Ossi recently told me her trick for a deep-flavored vegetarian broth (pictured on page 30) – she adds prunes to it. I'm telling you, it works! You can keep the vegetables left over from making stock and serve them deep-fried, or even as they are, with mayonnaise or aioli.

Serves 4

**Broth**

3 tbsp olive oil

3 carrots, peeled and cut into sticks

5 celery stalks, cut into chunks

1 large onion, quartered

½ celeriac, peeled and roughly chopped

7 garlic cloves, peeled

5 thyme sprigs

2 small bunches of parsley, plus some chopped parsley to garnish

10 black peppercorns

3 bay leaves

8 prunes

**Dumplings**

½ lb russet potato (1 small), peeled and diced

1½ cups peeled and diced parsnips

1 garlic clove, peeled

2 tbsp butter

½ cup self-rising flour (see note)

⅓ cup semolina

1 egg

salt and white pepper

To make the broth. Heat up the olive oil in a large pot. Add all the vegetables and garlic and sauté for a few minutes until they color lightly. Add the herbs, spices and prunes and cover with cold water. Simmer for up to 1½ hours, skimming the surface and adding more water when needed so that at the end of the cooking you are left with enough liquid for four portions.

Strain the broth through a fine sieve into a clean pan. Add some of the carrots and some celery or celeriac, if you like. Set aside ready for reheating.

To make the dumplings. Cook the potato, parsnips and garlic in plenty of boiling salted water until soft; drain well. Wipe dry the pan in which the vegetables were cooked and put them back inside. Add the butter and sauté on medium heat for a few minutes to get rid of the excess moisture. While hot mash them with a potato ricer or masher. Add the flour, semolina, egg, and some salt and pepper and mix until incorporated. Chill for 30 to 60 minutes, covered with plastic wrap.

Reheat the broth and taste for seasoning. In another pan, bring some salted water to a light simmer. Dip a teaspoon into the water and use it to spoon out the dumpling mix into the water. Once the dumplings come up to the surface, leave to simmer for 30 seconds, then remove from the water with a slotted spoon.

Ladle the hot broth into bowls. Place the dumplings in the broth, garnish with parsley and serve immediately.

Note: To make self-rising flour, combine 1 cup flour, 1¼ tsp baking powder, and a pinch of salt.

# Seasonal tempura

Here's the perfect solution for *all* your vegetables. This tempura (pictured on page 31) is breathtakingly delicious.

Serves 4
**Dipping sauce**
6 cardamom pods
grated zest and juice of 4 limes (about
⅓ cup juice)
1 fresh green chile
2¾ cups cilantro (leaves and stalks)
1 tbsp sugar
4 tbsp sunflower oil
½ tsp salt
2 tbsp water

About 2¾ lbs (net weight) freshly
prepared vegetables (see method),
such as: Jerusalem artichoke, beet,
broccoli, potato, sweet potato,
carrot, cauliflower, celeriac, baby
leek, parsnip, kohlrabi, salsify, turnip
½ cup cornstarch, plus extra to coat
the vegetables
½ cup self-rising flour (see note, facing
page)
¾ cup seltzer or sparkling water
2 tsp grapeseed oil
¼ tsp salt
chile flakes to taste
3 cups sunflower oil for deep-frying

To make the sauce. Break the cardamom pods using a mortar and pestle and transfer the seeds to a food-processor bowl. Discard the pods. Add the rest of the ingredients and blitz to get a smooth, runny sauce.

Next prepare the vegetables. There aren't any strict rules you must follow but try to keep them chunky and retain some of the natural shape of the vegetable where possible – for example, round vegetables cut into thin wedges and long ones into batons or strips. Here are a few useful suggestions. For cauliflower and broccoli, divide into medium florets; for beets, peel and cut into ⅛-inch-thick slices or wedges; for potatoes and sweet potatoes, leave the skin on and cut into ¼-inch-thick slices; for Jerusalem artichoke, carrot, parsnip, salsify, turnip and celeriac, peel and cut into ⅜-inch-thick sticks, not too perfect; for baby leeks just trim off the green ends.

Before you start frying the vegetables, prepare a large plate lined with paper towels. Scatter some cornstarch for coating the vegetables on another plate. Place the batter ingredients – flour, cornstarch, soda water, grapeseed oil and salt – in a bowl and whisk well to get a smooth, runny mix. Add some chile flakes for heat.

Pour the frying oil into a medium saucepan and place on high heat. Once very hot, turn the heat down to medium. When frying the vegetables, the oil should be hot enough so you get a good sizzle but not so hot that they burn.

Deep-fry four or five pieces of vegetable at a time. Take each piece and toss it in the cornstarch. Shake to remove any excess, then dip in the batter. Lift and shake again, then carefully put into the oil. As they fry, turn the pieces over to color evenly. Soft vegetables like leek should take about 1 minute to cook, harder ones like beets 2 minutes or more. When frying, occasionally remove any burnt bits that float in the oil. As they cook, transfer the vegetables onto the paper towels and keep warm.

When all the vegetables are cooked, serve them at once, with the dipping sauce on the side.

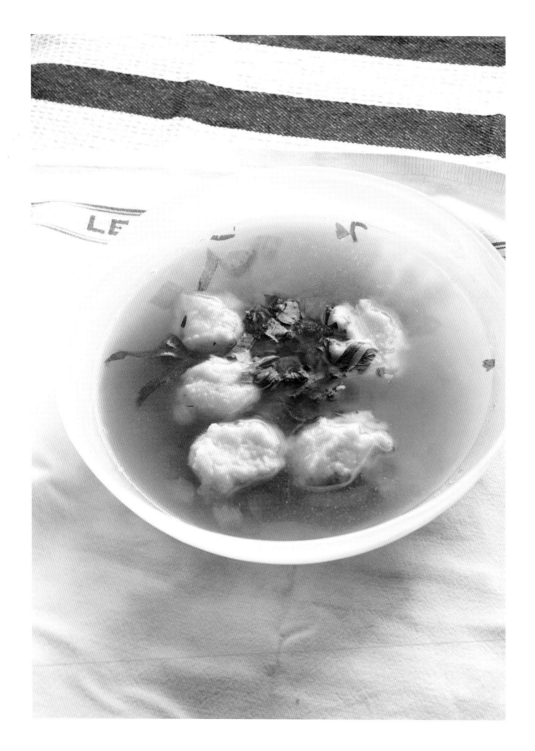

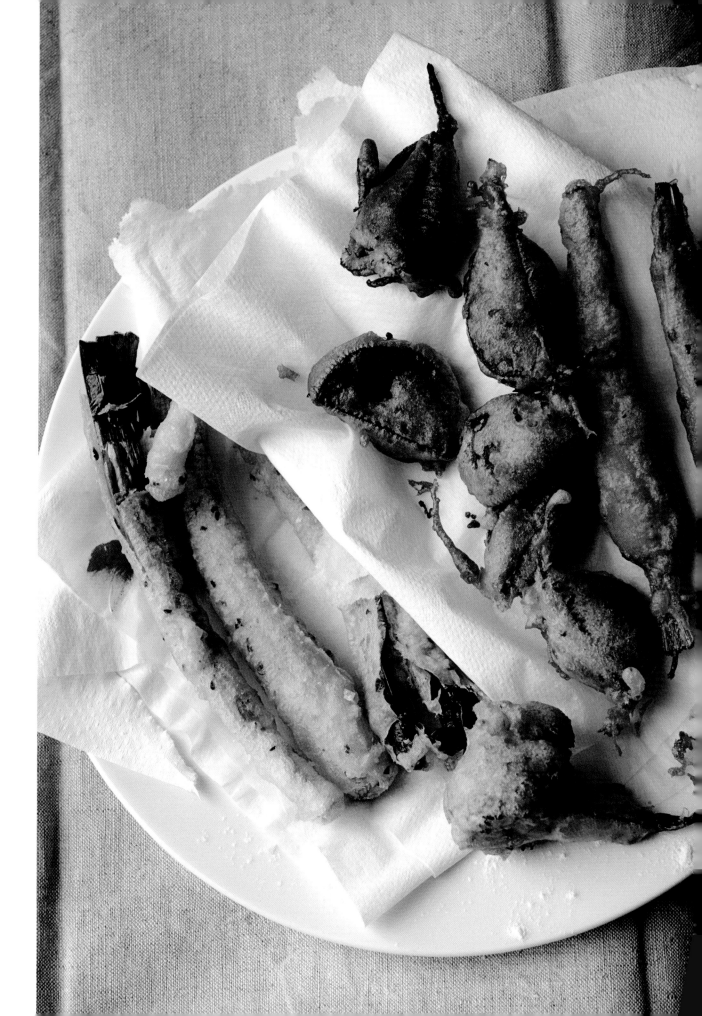

# Sweet potato cakes

When I was a student in Tel Aviv in the early 1990s I lived in the trendy center of the city, around Shenkin Street, and used to hang about in cafés with other students who, just like me, talked about meaningful things with an air of innocent self-importance. At the very heart of the center was a small café, called Orna and Ella's, that epitomized the scene; everyone wanted to be seen there. And what symbolized Orna and Ella's was their legendary sweet potato cakes. Here's a modified version.

Serves 4
2¼ lbs peeled sweet potatoes, cut into
   large chunks

Sauce
3 tbsp Greek yogurt
3 tbsp sour cream
2 tbsp olive oil
1 tbsp lemon juice
1 tbsp chopped cilantro
salt and black pepper

2 tsp soy sauce
scant ¾ cup all-purpose flour
1 tsp salt
½ tsp sugar
3 tbsp chopped green onion
½ tsp finely chopped fresh red chile
   (or more if you want them hot)
plenty of butter for frying

Steam the sweet potatoes until completely soft, then leave in a colander to drain for at least an hour.

To make the sauce. Whisk together all the sauce ingredients until smooth; set aside.

Once the sweet potatoes have lost most of their liquid, place them in a mixing bowl and add the rest of the ingredients (except the butter). Mix everything together, preferably by hand, until the mix is smooth and even; do not over-mix. The mixture should be sticky; if it's runny add some more flour.

Melt some butter in a non-stick frying pan. For each cake, use a tablespoon to lift some mix into the pan and flatten with the back of the spoon to create a not-too-perfect disc that is roughly 2 inches in diameter and ⅜ inch thick. Fry the cakes on medium heat for about 6 minutes on each side, or until you get a nice brown crust. Place in between two sheets of paper towels to soak up the excess butter. Serve hot or warm, with the sauce on the side.

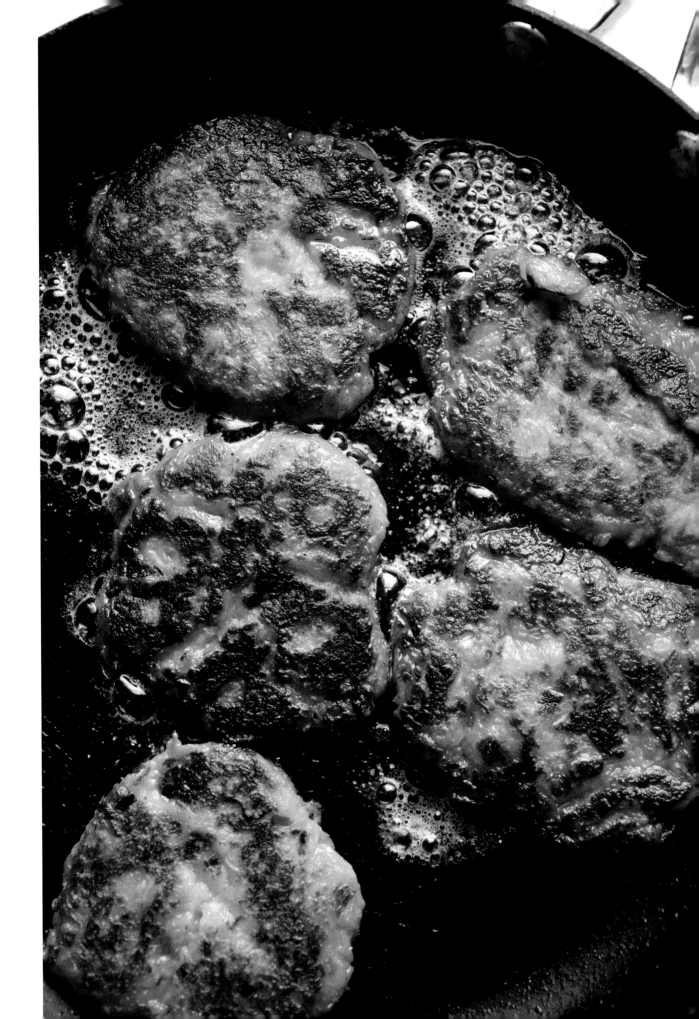

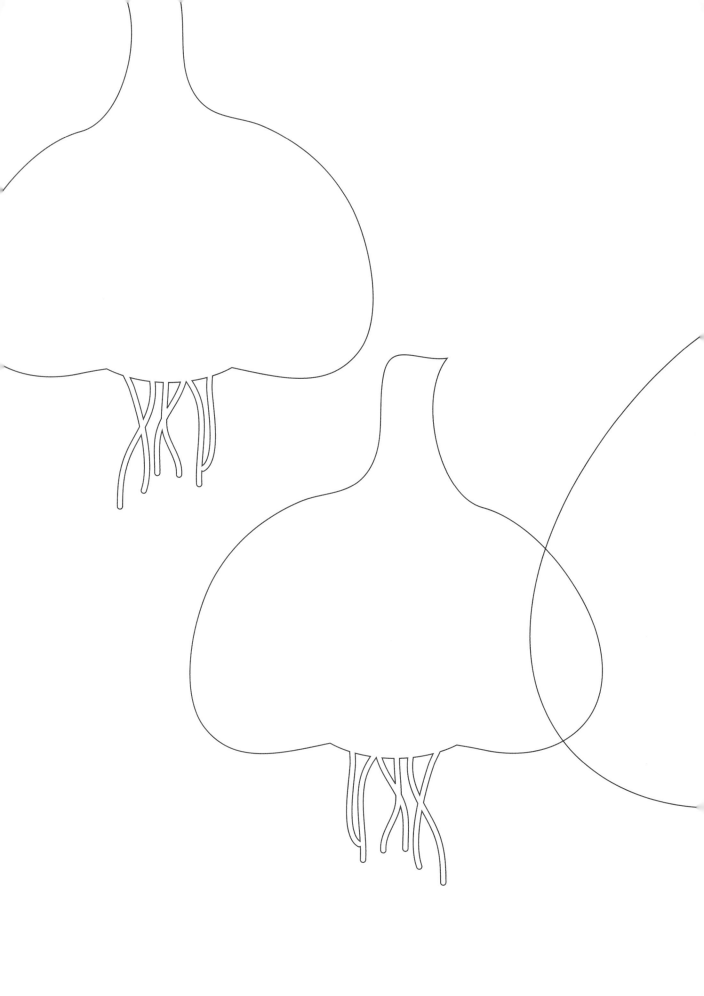

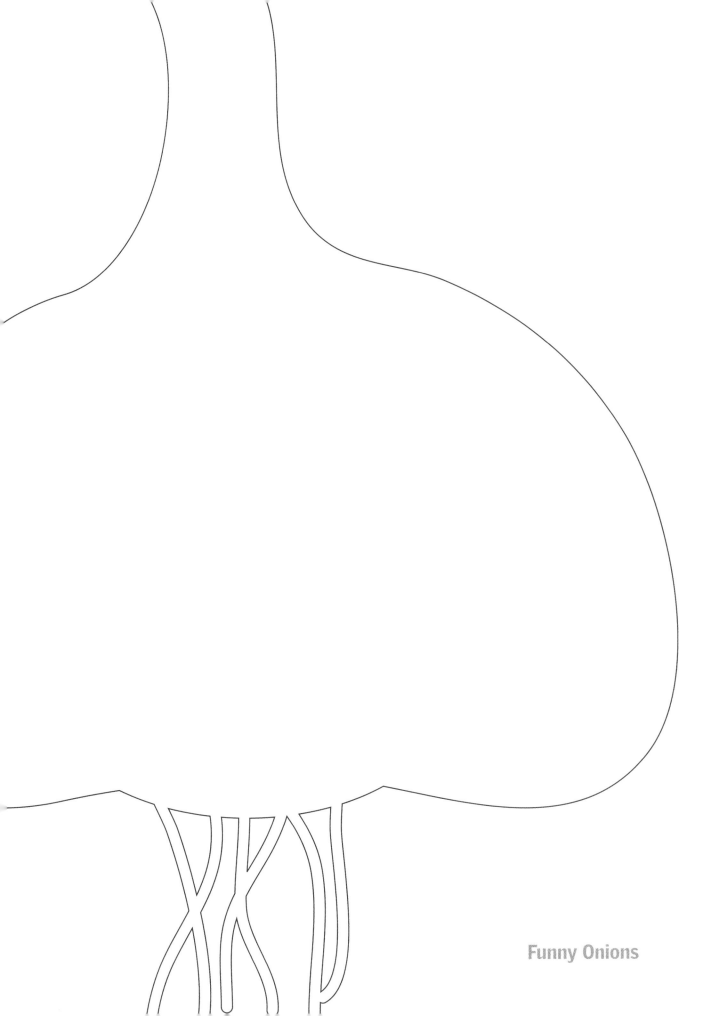

Funny Onions

# Leek fritters

My aunt, Yona Ashkenazi, makes the most heavenly leek fritters, inspired by her late husband Yaacov's Turkish descent. I have to admit I haven't eaten her wonderful food for many years but these fritters in particular, and another version made with spinach, remain distinct and sweet childhood memories. I believe my leek fritters come quite close.

Don't be put off by the long list of ingredients. You are likely to find many of them in your kitchen cupboard. You also don't *have* to make the sauce. A squirt of lemon or lime juice will suffice.

Serves 4

**Sauce**

½ cup Greek yogurt

½ cup sour cream

2 garlic cloves, crushed

2 tbsp lemon juice

3 tbsp olive oil

½ tsp salt

½ cup parsley leaves, chopped

2 cups cilantro leaves, chopped

3 leeks (1 lb in total, trimmed weight)

5 shallots, finely chopped

⅔ cup olive oil

1 fresh red chile, seeded and sliced

½ cup parsley (leaves and fine stalks), finely chopped

¾ tsp ground coriander

1 tsp ground cumin

¼ tsp ground turmeric

¼ tsp ground cinnamon

1 tsp sugar

½ tsp salt

1 egg white

¾ cup plus 1 tbsp self-rising flour (see page 28)

1 tbsp baking powder

1 egg

⅔ cup milk

4½ tbsp unsalted butter, melted

To make the sauce. Blitz all the ingredients together in a food processor until a uniform green. Set aside for later.

Cut the leeks into scant 1-inch-thick slices; rinse and drain dry. Sauté the leeks and shallots in a pan with half the oil on medium heat for about 15 minutes, or until soft. Transfer to a large bowl and add the chile, parsley, spices, sugar and salt. Allow to cool down.

Whisk the egg white to soft peaks and fold it into the vegetables. In another bowl mix together the flour, baking powder, whole egg, milk and butter to form a batter. Gently mix it into the egg white and vegetable mixture.

Put 2 tablespoons of the remaining oil in a large frying pan and place over a medium heat. Spoon about half of the vegetable mixture into the pan to make four large fritters. Fry them for 2 to 3 minutes on each side, or until golden and crisp. Remove to paper towels and keep warm. Continue making the fritters, adding more oil as needed. You should end up with about eight large fritters. Serve warm, with the sauce on the side or drizzled over.

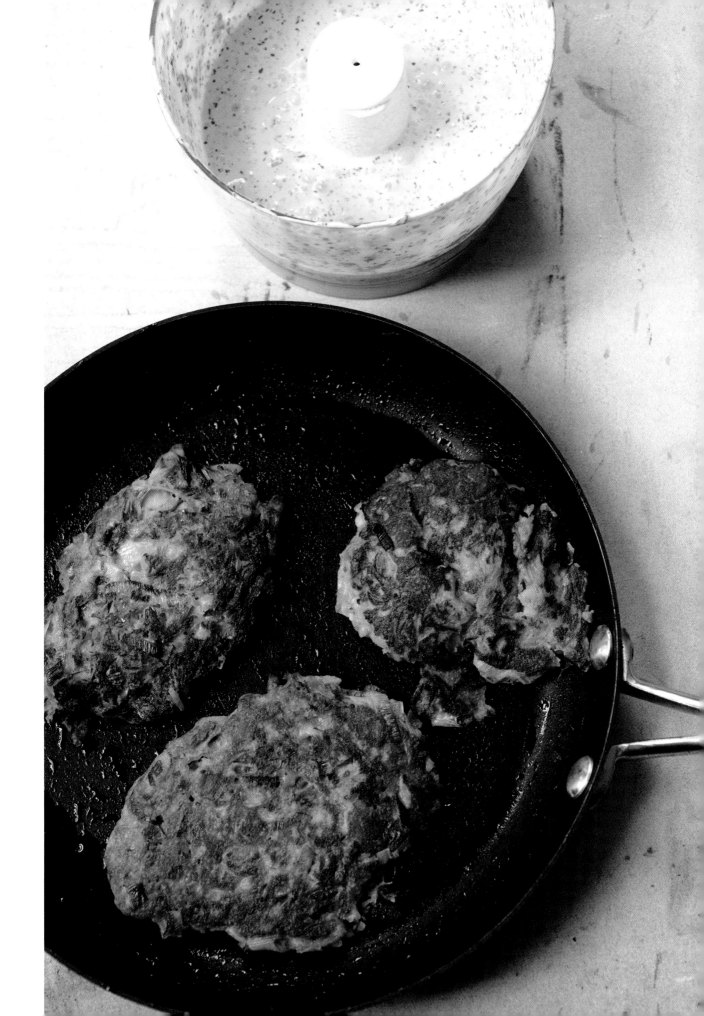

# Caramelized garlic tart

"I think this is the most delicious recipe (pictured on page 40) in the world!" wrote Claudine after trying it out for me. What else can I add?

Serves 8
13 oz puff pastry
3 medium heads of garlic, cloves
    separated and peeled
1 tbsp olive oil
1 tsp balsamic vinegar
1 cup water
¾ tbsp sugar
1 tsp chopped rosemary
1 tsp chopped thyme, plus a few whole
    sprigs to finish
salt
4½ oz soft, creamy goat cheese (such
    as chèvre)
4½ oz hard, mature goat cheese (such
    as goat gouda)
2 eggs
6½ tbsp heavy cream
6½ tbsp crème fraîche
black pepper

Have ready a shallow, loose-bottomed, 11-inch fluted tart pan. Roll out the puff pastry into a circle that will line the bottom and sides of the pan, plus a little extra. Line the pan with the pastry. Place a large circle of waxed paper on the bottom and fill up with pie weights or dried beans. Leave to rest in the fridge for about 20 minutes.

Preheat the oven to 350°F. Place the tart shell in the oven and blind bake for 20 minutes. Remove the weights and paper, then bake for 5 to 10 minutes more, or until the pastry is golden. Set aside. Leave the oven on.

While the tart shell is baking, make the caramelized garlic. Put the cloves in a small saucepan and cover with plenty of water. Bring to a simmer and blanch for 3 minutes, then drain well. Dry the saucepan, return the cloves to it and add the olive oil. Fry the garlic cloves on high heat for 2 minutes. Add the balsamic vinegar and water and bring to the boil, then simmer gently for 10 minutes. Add the sugar, rosemary, chopped thyme and ¼ teaspoon salt. Continue simmering on a medium flame for 10 minutes, or until most of the liquid has evaporated and the garlic cloves are coated in a dark caramel syrup. Set aside.

To assemble the tart, break both types of goat cheese into pieces and scatter in the tart shell. Spoon the garlic cloves and syrup evenly over the cheese. In a jug whisk together the eggs, cream, crème fraîche, ½ teaspoon salt and some black pepper. Pour this custard over the tart filling to fill the gaps, making sure that you can still see the garlic and cheese over the surface.

Reduce the oven temperature to 325°F and place the tart inside. Bake for 35 to 45 minutes, or until the tart filling has set and the top is golden brown. Remove from the oven and leave to cool a little. Then take out of pan, trim the pastry edge if needed, lay a few sprigs of thyme on top and serve warm (it reheats well!) with a crisp salad.

# Stuffed onions

This is an unusual yet delectable main course where the flavorful filling takes center stage. Consider creating a variation by spooning over a light tomato sauce before baking and sprinkling with cheese toward the end. Serve the onions (pictured on page 41) warm with a Lettuce Salad (page 146). I desperately urge you not to waste the flavored stock and onion cores; cook them together to make a base for a hearty onion soup.

Serves 4

butter for greasing the dish
2¼ cups vegetable stock
1½ cups white wine
4 large onions
3 small tomatoes
2⅔ cups fresh white breadcrumbs
3¼ oz feta, crumbled
1⅓ cups parsley leaves (loosely packed), finely chopped
3 tbsp olive oil, plus extra to finish
2 garlic cloves, crushed
3 green onions, thinly sliced
¾ tsp salt
black pepper

Preheat the oven to 350°F. Have ready a small buttered ovenproof dish.

Place the stock and white wine in a medium saucepan and bring to the boil. Meanwhile, trim ¼ inch off the top and bottom of the onions. Cut them lengthways in half and remove the brown skin. Gently remove most of the insides (keep these for another use), retaining two or three of the outer layers. Carefully separate the outer layers from each other and place them in the simmering stock, a few at a time. Cook for 3 to 4 minutes, or until just tender. Drain well and cool slightly. Keep the stock.

Use a coarse cheese grater to grate the tomatoes (you'll be left with most of the skin in your hand; discard it). Place the grated tomato in a large bowl and add the breadcrumbs, feta, parsley, olive oil, garlic, green onions, salt and some pepper.

Fill each onion layer generously with stuffing. Pull the sides together so you end up with a fat cigar shape. Place the stuffed onions, seam-side down, in the buttered dish and pour over about ⅓ cup of the reserved stock, just to cover the bottom of the dish. Bake for 45 to 50 minutes, or until the onions are soft and lightly colored and the stuffing is bubbling; add more stock if they dry completely before the end of the cooking process. Drizzle with oil and serve warm.

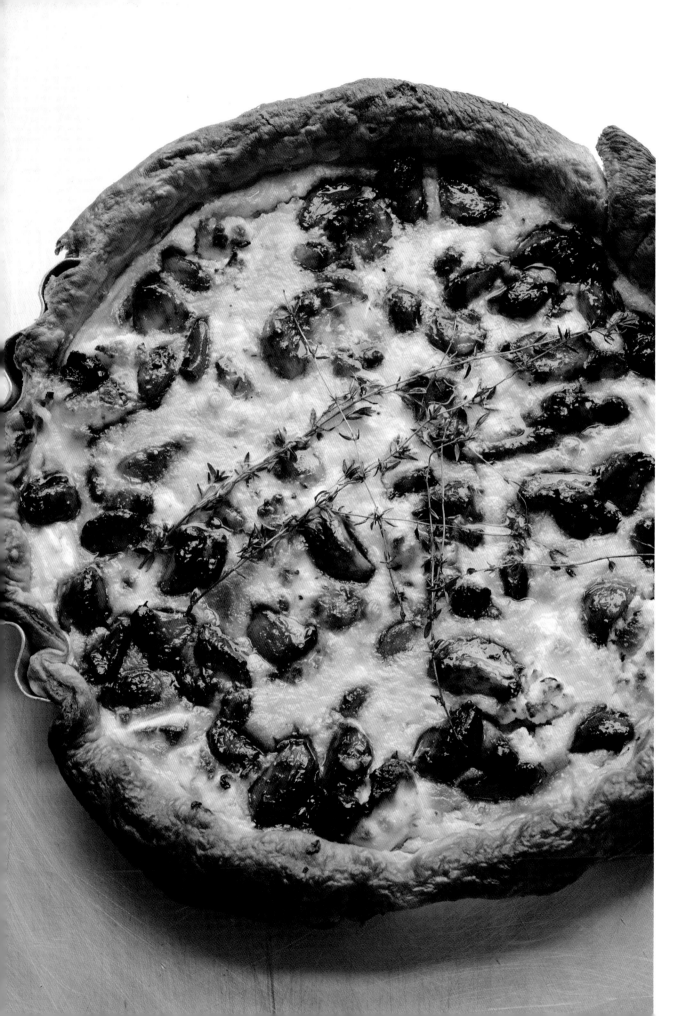

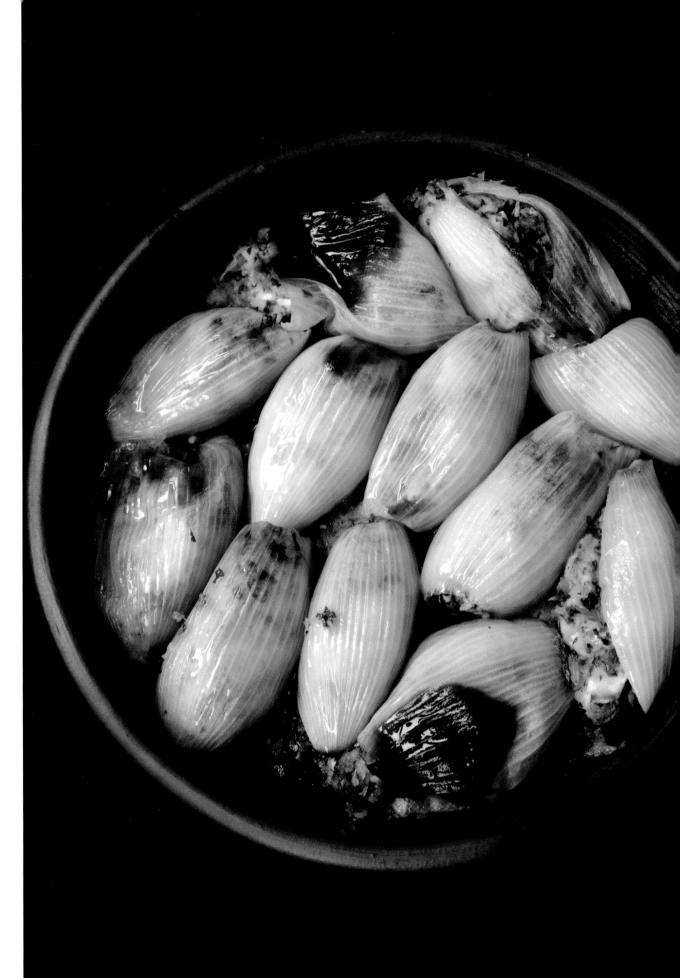

# Fried leeks

The sharp and sweet pickled red peppers used here are the sort of thing you can always keep in the fridge, ready to add to salads, roasted vegetables or salsas for fish.

Serves 4 as a starter
1 red bell pepper
6 tbsp sugar
1 cup water
6½ tbsp cider vinegar
10 pink peppercorns
½ tsp coriander seeds
3 cardamom pods, crushed
salt
5 medium leeks
¾ cup crème fraîche
1½ tbsp chopped capers
2 green onions, sliced thinly at an angle,
    plus extra to garnish
1 tbsp lemon juice
1½ tbsp olive oil
white pepper
⅔ cup sunflower oil
½ cup panko
1 egg, beaten

Clean the pepper and cut it into ¼-inch-thick strips. Place in a small saucepan and add the sugar, water, vinegar, peppercorns, coriander seeds, cardamom and some salt. Bring to the boil, then simmer for about 20 minutes, or until the pepper is cooked. Set aside to cool down.

Meanwhile, remove and discard the hard green leaves from the leeks and cut them into roughly 1-inch-long segments. Cook in boiling salted water for 15 minutes, or until semi-soft. Drain and let dry.

While you wait for the vegetables, stir together the crème fraîche, capers, green onions, lemon juice, olive oil and some salt and pepper. Taste and adjust the seasoning.

Heat up the sunflower oil in a medium saucepan. Place the panko and egg in two small separate plates and season with salt. Take the cooked leeks and roll them first in the egg and then in panko to coat all over. Fry them in the hot oil for about 30 seconds on each side; do this in a few batches so you don't crowd them in the pan. Once they are nice and golden, transfer the leeks to paper towels.

Serve about five chunks of hot leeks per portion, topped with a good dollop of the crème fraîche sauce. Lift the strips of red pepper out of the pan, shake away most of the syrup and place them over the leeks (the coriander seeds and peppercorns are fine too). Garnish with green onion and serve at once.

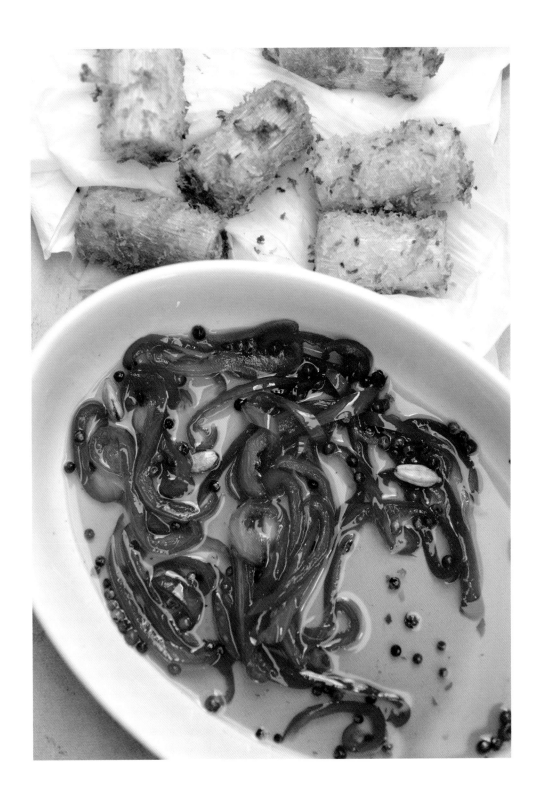

# Black pepper tofu

You will definitely surprise yourself with this one. It is an extremely delicious dish that's quick and straight-forward to make, but looks as if it's been prepared at a top Chinese restaurant. It is fiery, both from the chiles and the black pepper; you can moderate this by reducing their quantity a little. However, the whole point is spiciness so don't go too far.

Serves 4

1¾ lbs firm tofu

vegetable oil for frying

cornstarch to dust the tofu

11 tbsp butter

12 small shallots (12 oz in total), thinly sliced

8 fresh red chiles (fairly mild ones), thinly sliced

12 garlic cloves, crushed

3 tbsp chopped fresh ginger

3 tbsp sweet soy sauce (*kecap manis*)

3 tbsp light soy sauce

4 tsp dark soy sauce

2 tbsp sugar

5 tbsp coarsely crushed black peppercorns (use a mortar and pestle or a spice grinder)

16 small and thin green onions, cut into 1¼-inch segments

Start with the tofu. Pour enough oil into a large frying pan or wok to come ¼ inch up the sides and heat. Cut the tofu into large cubes, about 1 x 1 inch. Toss them in some cornstarch and shake off the excess, then add to the hot oil. (You'll need to fry the tofu pieces in a few batches so they don't stew in the pan.) Fry, turning them around as you go, until they are golden all over and have a thin crust. As they are cooked, transfer them onto paper towels.

Remove the oil and any sediment from the pan, then put the butter inside and melt it. Add the shallots, chiles, garlic and ginger. Sauté on low to medium heat for about 15 minutes, stirring occasionally, until the ingredients have turned shiny and are totally soft. Next, add the soy sauces and sugar and stir, then add the crushed black pepper.

Add the tofu to warm it up in the sauce for about a minute. Finally, stir in the green onions. Serve hot, with steamed rice.

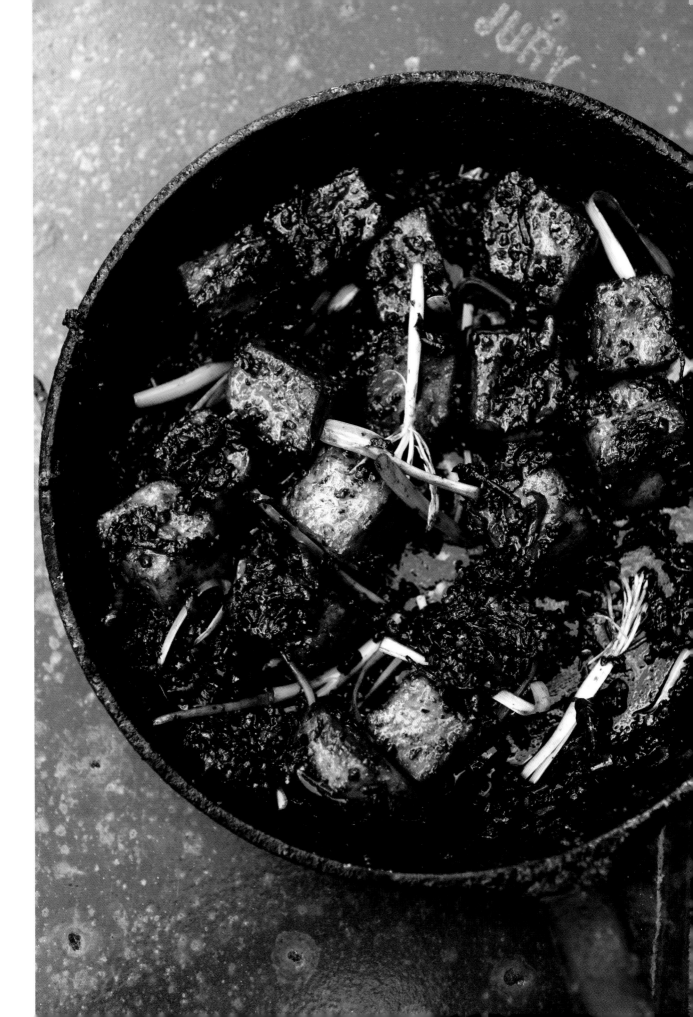

# Garlic soup and harissa

This soup is sweetly delicious and relatively easy to prepare, if you don't mind a bit of garlic peeling. The harissa adds work but you could substitute a good commercial variety. Still, this one makes a fantastic condiment to keep in your fridge and add to roasted eggplant, vegetable stews and many rice and couscous dishes.

Serves 4

**Harissa**

1 red bell pepper
¼ tsp coriander seeds
¼ tsp cumin seeds
¼ tsp caraway seeds
½ tbsp olive oil
1 small red onion, roughly chopped
3 garlic cloves, roughly chopped
2 medium–hot fresh red chiles,
    seeded and roughly chopped
½ tbsp tomato paste
2 tbsp lemon juice
⅔ tsp coarse sea salt

4 medium shallots, finely chopped
3 celery stalks, finely diced
3 tbsp butter
2 tbsp olive oil
25 medium garlic cloves, finely sliced
2 tsp chopped fresh ginger
1 tsp finely chopped thyme
1 cup white wine
generous pinch of saffron threads
4 bay leaves
1 quart good-quality vegetable stock
½ tsp coarse sea salt
4 tbsp roughly chopped parsley
roughly chopped cilantro
Greek yogurt (optional)

To make the harissa. Preheat the grill to high, then grill the bell pepper for 15 to 20 minutes, or until blackened all over. Transfer to a bowl, cover it with plastic wrap and allow to cool. Then peel the pepper and discard its seeds.

Place a frying pan on low heat and lightly dry-roast the coriander, cumin and caraway seeds for 2 minutes. Remove them to a mortar and use a pestle to grind to a powder.

Add the olive oil to the frying pan and heat, then fry the onion, garlic and chiles on medium heat for 6 to 8 minutes, to a dark smoky color. Cool slightly, then tip into a blender or a food processor. Add the remaining harissa ingredients, including the grilled pepper and ground spices, and blitz together to make a paste. Set aside.

Gently fry the shallots and celery with the butter and oil for about 10 minutes, or until soft and translucent. Add the garlic and cook for a further 5 minutes. Stir in the ginger and thyme. Pour in the wine and leave to simmer for a few minutes, then add the saffron, bay leaves, stock and salt. Simmer for about 10 minutes.

Remove the bay leaves and add the parsley. Blitz with an immersion blender (or regular blender) or a food processor. Do not blend to a complete purée; keep some bits of vegetable for texture.

Divide the soup among shallow bowls. Swirl in some harissa and sprinkle with chopped cilantro. Finish with a dollop of Greek yogurt, if you like.

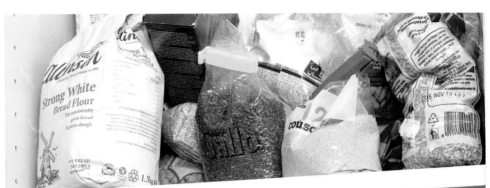

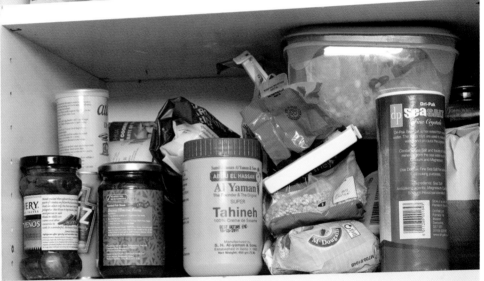

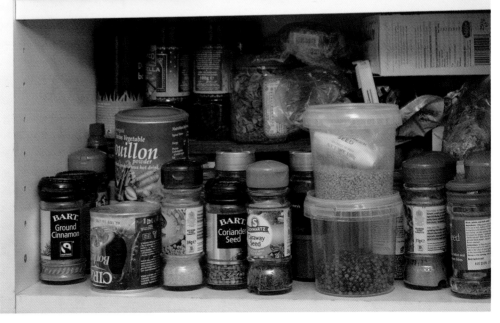

Mushrooms

# Mushroom ragout with poached duck egg

Here is my ideal solace for a gloomy winter night, even without the egg if you want to keep it simpler. If you can get fresh porcini (also called ceps), available during the autumn months, grab them with both hands and use as part of the mixed fresh mushrooms here.

Serves 4

½ oz dried porcini mushrooms

2½ cups water

1¼ lbs mixed fresh mushrooms (wild or cultivated)

¾ lb sourdough bread, crusts removed

6½ tbsp olive oil

2 garlic cloves, crushed

1 medium onion, sliced

1 medium carrot, peeled and sliced

3 celery stalks, sliced

½ cup white wine

3 thyme sprigs

salt

4 duck eggs

vinegar for poaching

½ cup sour cream

2 tbsp chopped tarragon

2 tbsp chopped parsley

black pepper

truffle oil (or olive oil if you prefer)

Before you start, put the dried porcini to soak in 1 cup of the water for 30 minutes. Brush your fresh mushrooms to remove any soil, then cut up large ones or divide into clusters so you have a selection of whole mushrooms and large chunks. Preheat the oven to 400°F.

Cut the bread into 1-inch cubes. Toss them with 2 tablespoons of the oil, the garlic and salt. Spread out on a baking sheet and toast in the oven for 15 minutes, or until brown.

Next, pour 1 tablespoon of oil into a medium-sized heavy pan and heat well over medium-high heat. Add some of the fresh mushrooms and leave for 1 to 2 minutes, without stirring. Don't crowd the mushrooms in the pan. Once lightly browned, turn them over to cook for another minute. Remove from the pan and continue with more batches, adding oil as needed. Once all the mushrooms have been removed from the pan, add another tablespoon of oil and throw in the onion, carrot and celery. Sauté on medium heat for 5 minutes, without browning. Add the wine and let it bubble away for a minute.

Lift the porcini out of the soaking liquid, squeezing out the excess liquid. Add the soaking liquid to the pan, leaving behind any grit in the bowl. Add the remaining 1½ cups of water, the thyme and a little salt, then simmer gently for about 20 minutes, or until you are left with about 1 cup of liquid. Strain this stock and discard the vegetables; return the stock to the pan and set it aside.

To poach the eggs, fill a shallow saucepan with enough water for a whole egg to cook in. Add a splash of vinegar and bring to a rapid boil. Carefully break an egg into a small cup and gently pour it into the boiling water. Immediately remove the pan from the heat and set it aside. After 6 minutes the egg should be poached to perfection. Lift it out of the pan and into a bowl of warm water. Once all the eggs are done, dry them on paper towels.

While you are poaching the final egg, heat up the stock and add all the mushrooms, the sour cream, most of the chopped herbs (reserving some to garnish) and salt and pepper to taste. As soon as the mushrooms are hot, place about four croutons in each serving dish and top with mushrooms. Add an egg, the remaining herbs, a drizzle of truffle oil and some black pepper.

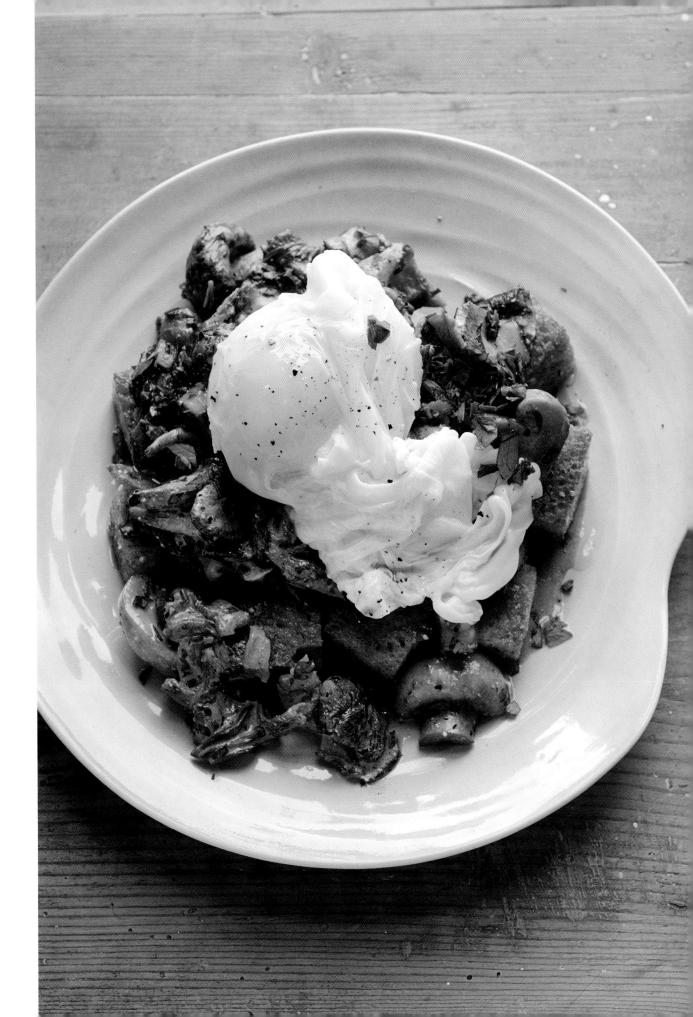

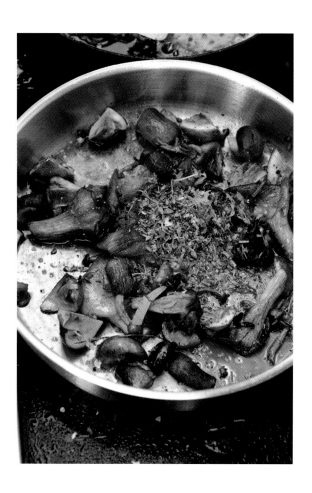

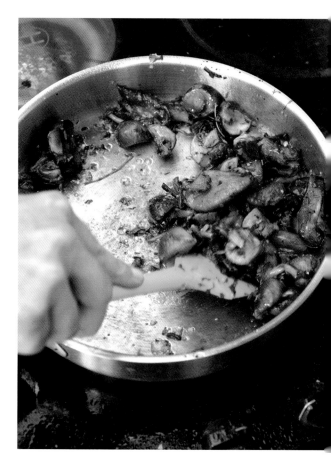

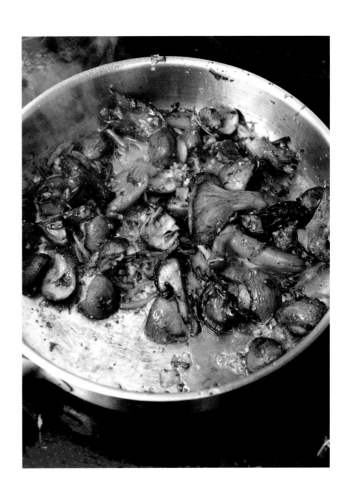

# Bánh xèo

In 2007 I visited Hanoi with my friend, Alex Meitlis, and found myself squatting in the dingiest of family-run street kitchens, experiencing the best food I've ever tasted. The freshness of the vegetables and herbs was mind-blowing.

Here's a vegetarian adaptation of a traditional Vietnamese pancake, normally consisting of fatty pork and prawns. I added sweet soy to the dipping sauce to make up for omitting the ubiquitous Vietnamese fish sauce, *nuoc mam*.

Serves 4
1⅓ cups rice flour
1 small egg
½ tsp salt
1 tsp ground turmeric
1¾ cups canned coconut milk
a little bit of sunflower oil

Sauce
2½ tbsp lime juice
1½ tbsp toasted sesame oil
1 tbsp brown sugar
1 tbsp rice wine vinegar
1 tbsp sweet soy sauce (*kecap manis*)
2 tsp grated fresh ginger
1 fresh red chile, finely chopped
1 garlic clove, crushed
½ tsp salt

Filling
1 large carrot, peeled
1 daikon radish, peeled
4 green onions
1 fresh green chile
1½ cups snow peas
1 cup loosely packed cilantro leaves
⅔ cup loosely packed Thai basil leaves
¼ cup loosely packed mint leaves
1 cup mung bean sprouts
1 cup enoki mushrooms

Blend the rice flour, egg, salt and turmeric in a large bowl. Slowly add the coconut milk, whisking well to avoid any lumps. You want to get a thinnish pancake batter with the consistency of light cream. Add more coconut milk or water, if necessary (you may need to add some more later, when you are cooking the pancakes, because the batter tends to thicken). Set aside to rest.

To make the sauce. Just whisk together all the ingredients, adjusting the amount of chile to your liking.

To make the filling. Shred the carrot and daikon thinly. Slice the green onions on an angle, and cut the green chile and snow peas into long, thin strips. Pick the herb leaves. Set all the prepared vegetables and herbs aside with the sprouts and mushrooms.

When you are ready to serve the pancakes, heat up a large non-stick frying pan that is roughly 9 inches in diameter, making sure it doesn't get extremely hot. Add a tiny amount of sunflower oil.

Pour in about one-quarter of the batter and swirl around to coat the bottom of the pan. The edges of the pancake can be thinner than the center and turn crisp, or it can all have the same thickness like a regular pancake. Once the underside is golden brown, turn the pancake over and cook the other side. Remove from the pan and keep warm while you make the other three pancakes.

Place a warm pancake on each serving plate and pile vegetables and herbs over one half of it. Drizzle the vegetables with some sauce and fold the other half of the pancake over them. Spoon some more sauce on top and serve, with any remaining sauce on the side.

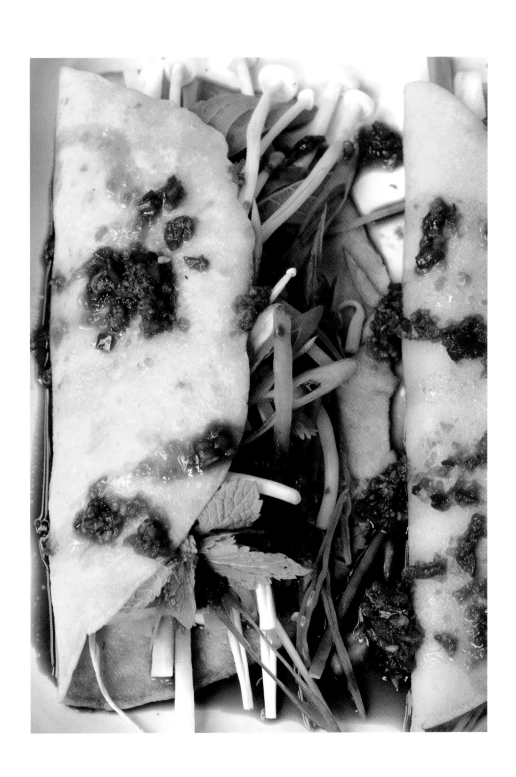

# Stuffed portobello with melting Taleggio

I can easily imagine someone writing a Ph.D. thesis on different cheeses and how they melt. Here are a few of my modest observations: young varieties, such as fontina or mozzarella, melt at a relatively low temperature and therefore don't "break" but stay creamy and smooth; other, more mature cheeses, such as Gruyère and some cheddars, are wonderfully pungent but tend to split and turn gritty. This is why I often choose Taleggio, a wonderfully soft cow's milk variety from northern Italy. It has the strong aroma of a mature cheese and melts evenly and smoothly.

Serves 4 as a starter

4 large portobellos (or another similar mushroom), stalks removed

6 tbsp olive oil

salt and black pepper

1 small onion, finely diced

1 celery stalk, finely diced

2 cups finely chopped sun-dried tomatoes

2 garlic cloves, crushed

½ cup grated Parmesan

1 tbsp chopped tarragon leaves

4 tbsp coarsely shredded basil leaves

3½ oz Taleggio, sliced

Preheat the oven to 350°F. Line a baking sheet with parchment paper. Place the mushrooms, stalk-side up, on the baking sheet and drizzle over a little oil and some salt and pepper. Put into the oven and roast for about 15 minutes, or until the mushrooms begin to soften.

Meanwhile, heat up 2 tablespoons of the oil in a sauté pan, add the onion and celery and cook on low heat for 5 to 10 minutes, or until the vegetables are soft but not brown; stir every few minutes during cooking. Add the sun-dried tomatoes and garlic and cook for a few more minutes. Remove from the heat and leave to cool down.

Once cool, add the Parmesan, tarragon and half the basil to the mixture and season with pepper. (You can add a little bit of salt but not too much because Taleggio is very salty.) Pile up the filling on the whole mushrooms and top with the Taleggio slices. Return to the oven and cook for about 10 minutes, or until the cheese melts and the mushrooms are tender.

Transfer the mushrooms to serving plates and drizzle with oil. Garnish with the remaining basil and serve right away, with a green salad.

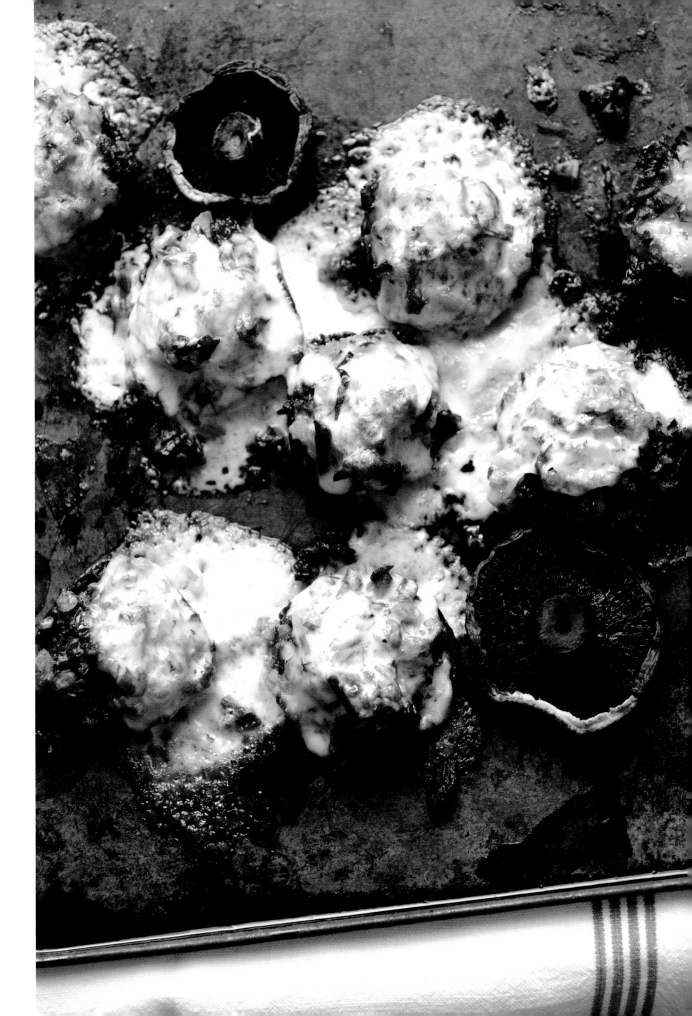

# Marinated mushrooms with walnut and tahini yogurt

This dish can work in endless contexts: with a few elegant endive leaves stirred through, it will make a substantial vegetarian main course; as it is you can put it in a Tupperware container and take it on a picnic; or offer it alongside other salads as part of a smart spring buffet.

Shimeji are the clustered small mushrooms that you often get in "exotic" selections.

Serves 4
⅓ cup olive oil
1 tbsp white wine vinegar
1 tbsp maple syrup
juice of 2 medium lemons
salt and black pepper
3 cups sliced button mushrooms
2 cups beech mushrooms, large base
    removed
½ cup Greek yogurt
2½ tbsp tahini
1 small garlic clove, crushed
3 cups shelled fava beans (frozen
    or fresh)
⅔ cup walnuts, toasted and roughly
    chopped
½ tsp ground cumin
1 tbsp chopped dill
1 tbsp chopped oregano

Start by marinating the mushrooms. Whisk together the olive oil, vinegar, maple syrup, half the lemon juice, about ½ teaspoon salt and some black pepper. Pour this over the mixed mushrooms in a large bowl and toss well, making sure all the mushrooms are coated. Leave them to marinate for an hour.

While you wait, mix together in a small bowl the yogurt, tahini, garlic, remaining lemon juice and ½ teaspoon salt. Use a fork or a small whisk to whip everything together to a light paste. (You can refrigerate this sauce for up to a day.)

Next, pour plenty of boiling water over the fava beans in a bowl and leave for a minute, then drain well and leave to cool down. Now squeeze each bean gently to remove the skin and discard it (if you don't mind the skin you can skip this stage).

Add the beans, walnuts and cumin to the marinated mushrooms and stir to mix. Taste and adjust the seasoning. Serve the mushrooms in small bowls or plates, each portion topped with a dollop of thick tahini sauce and sprinkled with herbs.

# Mushroom lasagne

It took the aid of *Cook's Illustrated*, a magazine for food nerds like me, to enable me to crack the secret for a perfect cheesy lasagne. Serve this with an arugula and tomato salad.

Serves 6–8

1¼ oz dried porcini mushrooms

1¾ cups lukewarm water

5 tbsp unsalted butter

1 tbsp thyme leaves

1¾ lbs mixed fresh mushrooms, sliced if large

2 tbsp chopped tarragon

4 tbsp chopped parsley

salt and white pepper

5 tbsp unsalted butter

1 small shallot, chopped

scant ½ cup all-purpose flour

2⅓ cups milk

13 fl oz ricotta

1 large egg

5 oz feta, crumbled

6 oz Gruyère, grated

1 lb dried spinach lasagne

5 oz fontina cheese (or mozzarella), grated

½ cup grated Parmesan

Preheat the oven to 350°F. Cover the porcini with the lukewarm water and leave to soak for 5 minutes. Drain in a sieve set over a bowl, squeezing the mushrooms to remove all the liquid; reserve the liquid.

Melt the butter in a large heavy-based saucepan. When foaming add the thyme, porcini and fresh mushrooms. Cook for 4 minutes, or until the mushrooms have softened and exuded some of their liquid, stirring occasionally. Off the heat, stir in the tarragon, parsley and some salt and pepper. Transfer to a bowl and set aside.

Use the same pan to make a béchamel. Put the butter and shallot in the pan and cook on medium heat for about a minute. Add the flour and continue cooking, stirring constantly, for 2 minutes; the mix will turn into a paste but shouldn't color much. Gradually whisk in the milk and porcini soaking liquid, leaving any grit in the bowl. Add ½ teaspoon salt and continue whisking until boiling. Simmer on low heat, stirring constantly, for about 10 minutes, or until the sauce is thickish. Remove from the heat.

In a small bowl mix together the ricotta and egg, then fold in 3 tablespoons of the béchamel and the feta. Add the Gruyère to the remaining béchamel in the pan and stir well to get your main sauce.

Pour boiling water over the lasagne noodles (do this a few at a time so they don't stick together) and soak for 2 minutes; remove and dry them on a tea towel.

To assemble the lasagne, pour one-fifth of the sauce over the bottom of an ovenproof dish that is about 10 x 14 inches. Cover with lasagne noodles. Spread one-quarter of the ricotta mix on top, scatter over one-quarter of the mushrooms and sprinkle with one-quarter of the fontina. Make three more layers in the same way, then finish with a layer of pasta covered with sauce.

Sprinkle the Parmesan on top and cover loosely with foil (don't lay it directly on the surface of the lasagne). Bake for 40 minutes, or until the sauce is bubbling around the sides. Lift off the foil and bake for a further 10 minutes, or until the top turns golden. Remove from the oven and leave to rest for 10 minutes before serving.

# Wild mushroom parcel

Cooking in a parcel, albeit a tad old-fashioned, is actually both simple and exciting. There is always an element of suspense when diners open their own little packet to a whiff of aromatic steam. Loads of herbs and tender baby vegetables are the perfect ingredients for this method, as are many kinds of fish.

Serve the mushrooms with a bowl of steamed white rice sprinkled with salted and toasted pine nuts or pumpkin seeds.

Serves 4
3½ cups mixed wild mushrooms
3½ cups baby button mushrooms
5 baby potatoes, cooked (skin on)
4 garlic cloves, crushed
8 tbsp chopped chervil
4 tbsp chopped tarragon
4 tbsp olive oil
8 tbsp heavy cream
2 tbsp Ricard, Pernod or other anise-
    flavored liquor
salt and black pepper

Preheat the oven to 400°F. Cut four square sheets of parchment paper 14 inches long and wide.

Wipe the mushrooms clean using a wet cloth or a little brush. Leave them whole or cut them into large pieces, depending on their size. Cut the potatoes into ⅜-inch-thick slices.

In a large bowl, gently toss together all of the ingredients using your hands. Take care not to break the mushrooms. Taste and adjust the amount of salt and pepper.

Divide the mix between the paper sheets. Lift the edges and scrunch them together to create tight bundles, then secure with ovenproof string. Lift the parcels onto a baking sheet.

Place in the oven to cook for 17 minutes. Take out and leave to settle for 1 minute. Serve the parcels sealed, allowing the diners to open them up themselves.

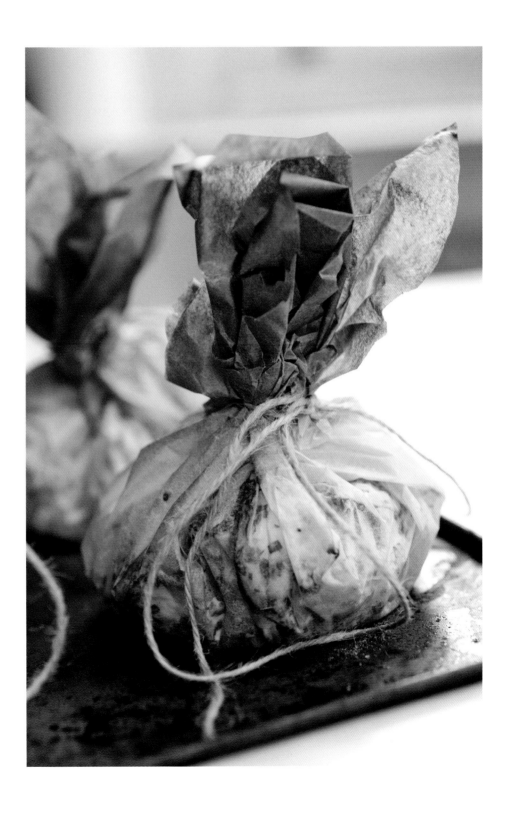

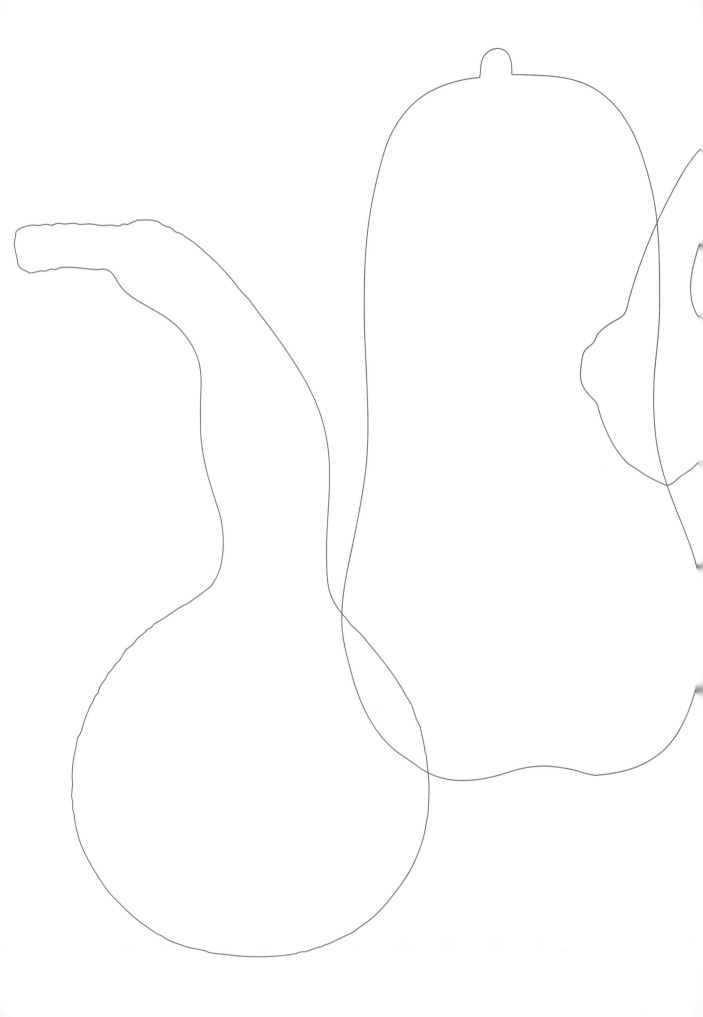

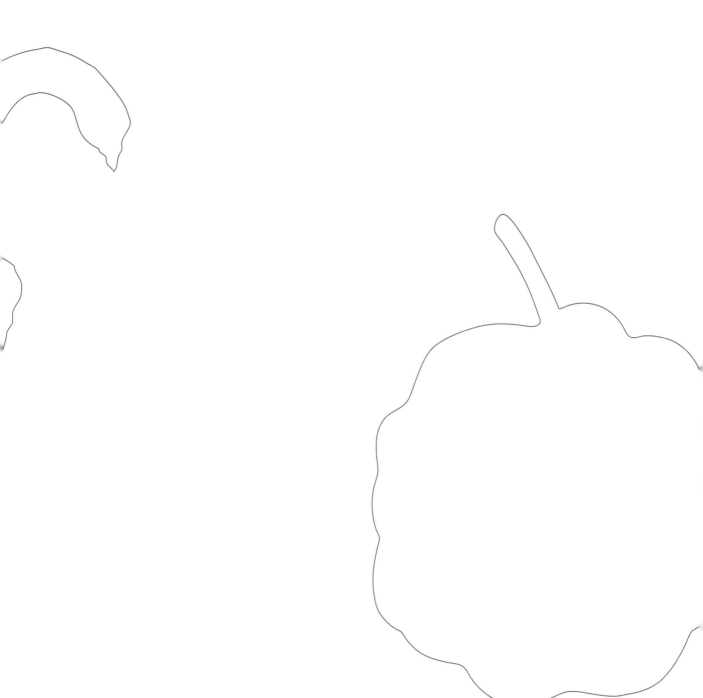

Zucchini and Other Squashes

# Halloween soufflés

To introduce this dish I reprise a famous supermarket's slogan: "Try something scary today." By scary I mean a soufflé, which is so many people's no-go zone. I've called them Halloween soufflés as they are made with pumpkin. It's best not to use one of those huge pumpkins destined to be jack-o'-lanterns as their flesh can be watery.

The soufflé base mixture, minus the egg whites, can be prepared a day in advance and kept in the fridge. Just bring it back to room temperature before finishing the recipe. These soufflés (pictured on page 66) look particularly striking in shallow soup bowls. If you have an ovenproof set, try using them.

Serves 6 in ramekins as a starter, or
    4 in soup bowls
one ¾-lb pumpkin (skin on)
olive oil
¾ tsp soft brown sugar
salt
¼ cup whole hazelnuts (skin on)
4 tbsp unsalted butter; 2 tbsp, melted,
    for greasing
2½ tbsp all-purpose flour
1 cup plus 1 tbsp milk
5 eggs, separated, plus one egg white
¼ tsp chile flakes
1 tbsp chopped marjoram
2½ oz strong goat cheese, grated
⅓ cup sour cream
2 tbsp chopped chives

Preheat the oven to 350°F. Depending on the size of the pumpkin, cut it into quarters or eighths. Scoop out and discard the seeds and fibers. Place the pumpkin pieces skin-side down in a shallow roasting tin. Drizzle over a little olive oil and sprinkle with the brown sugar and ½ teaspoon salt. Roast for 45 minutes, or until the flesh is tender. Leave to cool for a while, then scoop out the flesh and blitz it to a purée or mash well. You need exactly 4¼ oz for the soufflés.

Turn up the oven to 400°F and place a baking sheet on the top shelf. This will help with the rising when the soufflés are set on it. Put the ramekins or bowls in the fridge to chill well.

Blitz the hazelnuts in a blender or food processor until powdery. Brush the chilled ramekins generously with the melted butter, then put in the hazelnuts and turn the dishes to coat the bottom and sides. Tip out the excess nuts and set aside.

Melt the 2 tbsp butter in a large saucepan over a medium heat. Stir in the flour and cook for a minute. Gradually add the milk, stirring with a wooden spoon until the sauce is thick and starts to bubble. In a large bowl mix together the 4¼ oz pumpkin, egg yolks, chile flakes, marjoram, goat cheese and ¾ teaspoon salt. Add the sauce and stir until smooth.

Place the egg whites in a large, clean, stainless steel or glass bowl and whisk until they are stiff but not dry. Add a little of the egg whites to the pumpkin base and stir to loosen, then fold in the remaining egg whites with a large, stainless steel spoon, taking care to retain as much air as possible.

Fill the ramekins or bowls up to ⅜ inch from the top. Place the soufflés in the oven, on the heated baking sheet, and bake for 10 to 14 minutes, or until golden brown and risen well.

While they are in the oven, mix the sour cream with the chives. Serve the soufflés at once, with the sour cream on the side.

# Roasted butternut squash with sweet spices, lime and green chile

This dish (pictured on page 67) is the most refreshing way I can think of to start a meal.

Serves 4–6
2 limes
Maldon sea salt
4 tablespoons olive oil
1 medium butternut squash (about 2 lbs)
2 tbsp cardamom pods
1 tsp ground allspice
½ cup Greek yogurt
2½ tbsp tahini
1 tbsp lime juice
1 green chile, thinly sliced
⅔ cup picked cilantro leaves

Preheat the oven to 400°F. Trim off the limes' tops and bases using a small sharp knife. Stand each lime on a chopping board and cut down the sides of the fruit, following its natural curves, to remove the skin and white pith. Quarter the limes from top to bottom, and cut each quarter into thin slices, about ⅛ inch thick. Place them in a small bowl, sprinkle with a little salt, drizzle with 1 tablespoon of the olive oil, stir and set aside.

Next, cut the squash in half lengthways, scoop out the seeds and discard. Cut each half, top to bottom, into ⅜-inch-thick slices and lay them out on a large baking sheet lined with parchment paper.

Place the cardamom pods in a mortar and work with a pestle to get the seeds out of the pods. Discard the pods and work the seeds to a rough powder. Transfer to a small bowl, add the allspice and the remaining 3 tablespoons of oil, stir well and brush this mixture over the butternut slices. Sprinkle over a little salt and place in the oven for 15 minutes or until tender when tested with the point of a knife. Remove from the oven and set aside to cool. Peel off the skin, or leave on if you prefer.

Meanwhile, whisk together the yogurt, tahini, lime juice, 2 tablespoons of water and a pinch of salt. The sauce should be thick but runny enough to pour; add more water if necessary.

To serve, arrange the cooled butternut slices on a serving platter and drizzle with the yogurt sauce. Spoon over the lime slices and their juices and scatter the chile slices over the top. Garnish with the cilantro and serve.

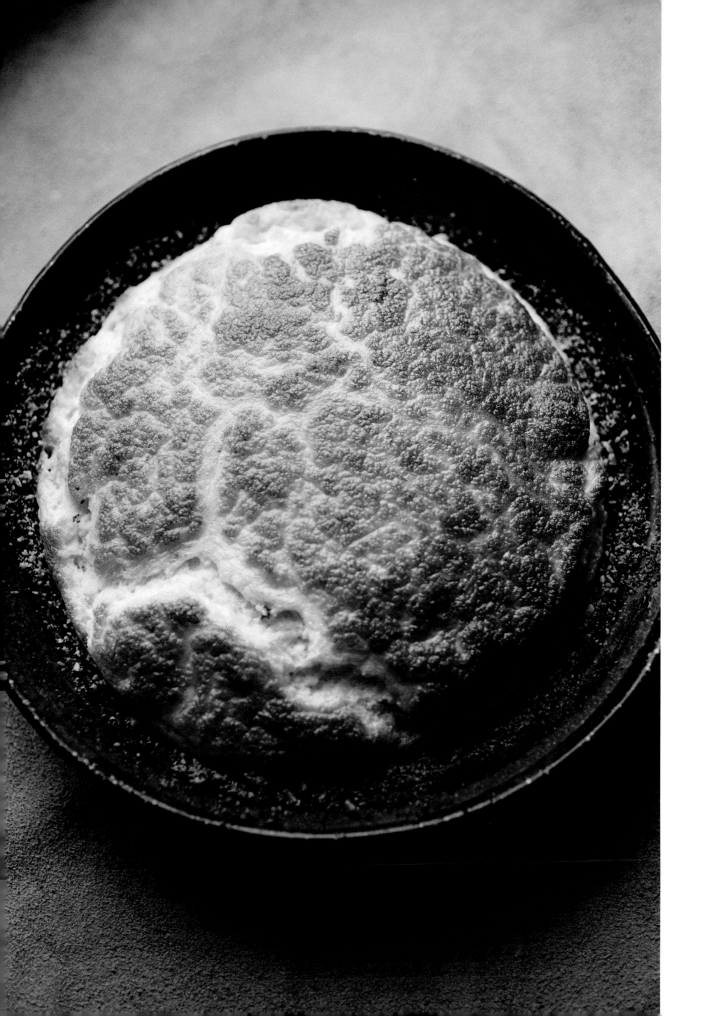

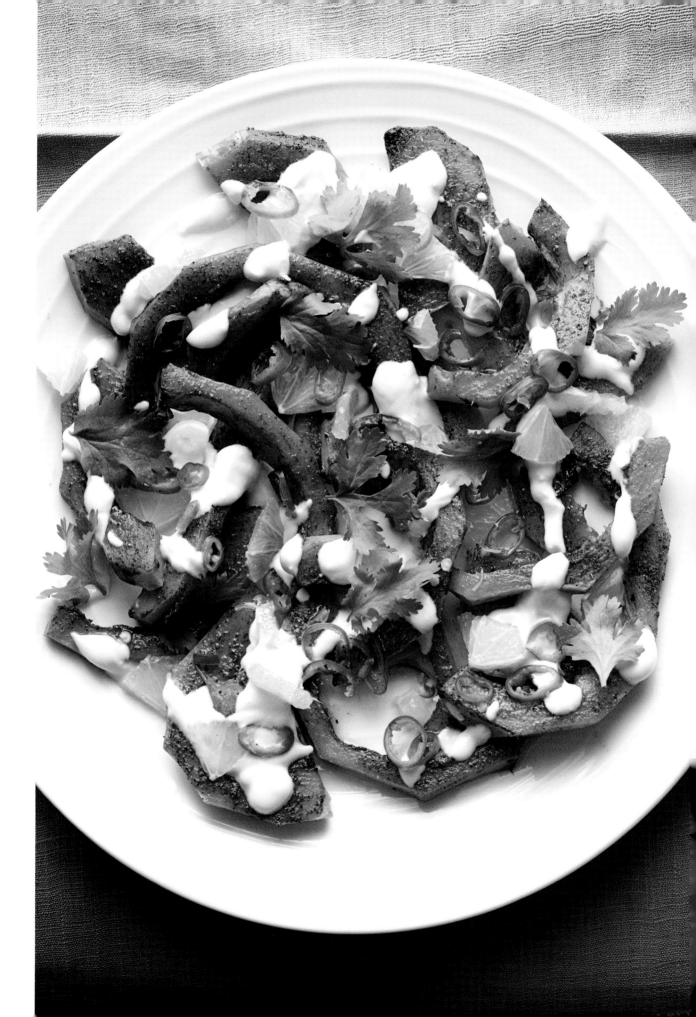

# "Mixed grill" with parsley oil

Char-grilling seasonal vegetables the way we often do at Ottolenghi makes them taste almost meaty due to the strong aromas of smoke and the many burnt bits. I just love it. You don't have to stick to my choice of vegetables. There are countless alternatives, such as asparagus, rutabaga, carrot, cauliflower, daikon, beets and so on.

Choose a soft cheese that won't disintegrate or melt on the grill, such as Greek manouri or Cypriot anari (handle it with care). They are available from Middle Eastern grocers (see Dates and Turkish Sheep's Cheese, page 280). Alternatively, use halloumi, but eat it while it's still warm, before it turns rubbery.

Serves 4 generously

**Parsley oil**

¾ cup flat-leaf parsley (leaves and
    soft stalks)
⅓ cup olive oil
2 garlic cloves, crushed
1½ tbsp lemon juice
salt and black pepper

1 medium zucchini
1 kohlrabi
1 small eggplant (or ½ medium)
4½ oz Manouri or anari cheese
3 to 4 tbsp olive oil

To make the parsley oil. Blitz the parsley in a food processor with the oil, garlic, lemon juice and some salt and pepper. You will get a bright green, runny sauce. Set it aside.

Place a heavy ridged griddle pan on a high heat and leave it until very hot. Preheat the oven to 375°F.

Cut the zucchini on a slight angle into ⅜-inch-thick slices. Peel the kohlrabi with a sharp knife; cut lengthways in half, then into ⅜-inch-thick slices. Slice the eggplant ¼ inch thick. Slice the cheese ¼ inch thick. Keeping all the ingredients separate, toss them in a little bit of olive oil (the eggplant will need much more oil as it readily soaks it up) and sprinkle with salt.

Char-grill the vegetables and cheese, in batches, until just tender and with nice char marks on both sides – they will take between 1 minute (the zucchini) and 6 minutes (the eggplant). Use tongs and a spatula to turn them. When done remove them to a mixing bowl, keeping the cheese separate. Transfer the eggplant to the hot oven to finish cooking through, 5 to 10 minutes more.

Pour the parsley oil over the hot vegetables and stir gently, then let them cool down completely or until warm.

Before serving, taste and adjust the seasoning. Spread the vegetables and the cheese on a platter and serve.

# Stuffed zucchini

This is a bastardized version of a Turkish original. Serve it cold, just above fridge temperature, with goat's-milk yogurt.

Serves 6 as a starter
1 medium onion, finely chopped
1 tbsp olive oil
⅔ cup short-grain rice
2 tbsp currants
1 tbsp pine nuts
2 tbsp chopped parsley, plus extra
    to garnish
½ tsp dried mint
½ tsp ground allspice
¼ tsp ground cinnamon
¼ tsp ground cloves
3 tbsp lemon juice
3 medium zucchini
¾ cup boiling water
1½ tbsp sugar
salt and black pepper

Sauté the onion in the oil until softened. Add the rice, currants, pine nuts, parsley, mint, spices and half the lemon juice. Continue cooking on low heat for 5 minutes, stirring occasionally.

Halve the zucchini lengthways along the center and use a spoon to scoop out some of the flesh to make "boats." Place them in a shallow saucepan that is large enough to accommodate them side by side. Fill them with the rice stuffing. Pour the boiling water, remaining lemon juice, sugar and some salt around the zucchini. The liquid should not come as high as the filling.

Simmer, covered, for 30 to 40 minutes, basting the filling occasionally with the cooking juices. The zucchini are ready when the rice is al dente and almost all the juices have evaporated. Allow to cool down completely before refrigerating. Garnish with chopped parsley when serving.

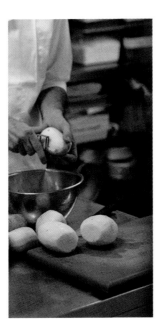

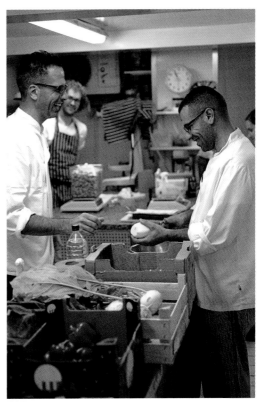

# Zucchini and hazelnut salad

Fresh hazelnuts are wonderfully sweet and juicy. They have a short season, from mid-August until October, but are worth using for this salad if you can get them. Try them first and decide for yourself whether you want to roast them as I describe, or keep fresh. With or without hazelnuts, this makes the most luxurious summer starter.

Serves 4

⅓ cup shelled hazelnuts

7 small zucchini (1¾ lbs in total)

4 tbsp olive oil

salt and black pepper

1 tsp balsamic vinegar

1¼ cups mixed green and purple basil leaves

3 oz top-quality Parmesan, broken up or very thinly sliced

2 tsp hazelnut oil

Preheat the oven to 300°F. Scatter the hazelnuts over a baking sheet and roast for 12 to 15 minutes, or until nicely browned. Let them cool down before chopping roughly or just crushing lightly with the side of a large knife.

Place a ridged griddle pan on a high heat and leave it there until it's almost red-hot – at least 5 minutes.

Meanwhile, trim the ends of the zucchini and cut them on an angle into ⅜-inch-thick slices. Place them in a bowl and toss with half the olive oil and some salt and pepper. Place the slices in the hot grill pan and char-grill for about 2 minutes on each side; turn them over using tongs. You want to get distinct char marks without cooking the zucchini through. Transfer to a mixing bowl, pour over the balsamic vinegar, toss together and set aside.

Once the zucchini have cooled down, add the remaining olive oil, the basil and hazelnuts. Mix lightly, then taste and adjust the seasoning accordingly. Transfer the salad to a flat plate, incorporating the Parmesan, and drizzle over the hazelnut oil.

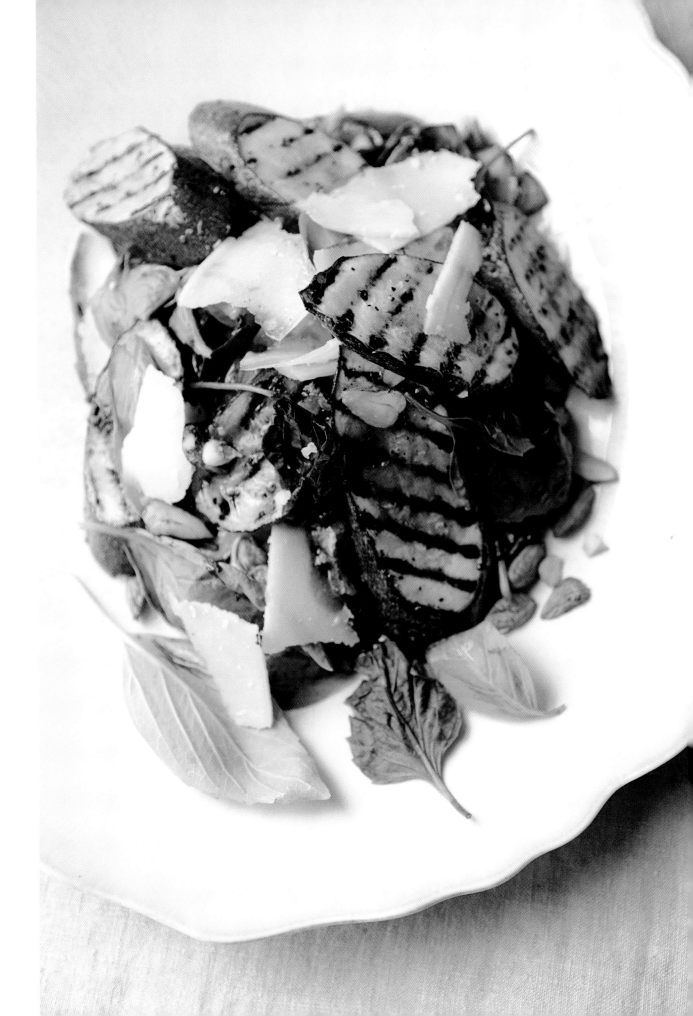

# Crusted pumpkin wedges with sour cream

You can use most varieties of pumpkin for these satisfying wedges. Serve with Green Gazpacho (page 180) to make a light and healthy-feeling supper. They will also make a perfect veggie main course for Christmas as the crust is a bit like stuffing.

Serves 4
1½ lbs pumpkin (skin on)
½ cup grated Parmesan
3 tbsp dried white breadcrumbs
6 tbsp finely chopped parsley
2½ tsp finely chopped thyme
grated zest of 2 large lemons
2 garlic cloves, crushed
salt and white pepper
¼ cup olive oil
½ cup sour cream
1 tbsp chopped dill

Preheat the oven to 375°F. Cut the pumpkin into ⅜-inch-thick slices and lay them flat, cut-side down, on a baking sheet that has been lined with parchment paper.

Mix together in a small bowl the Parmesan, breadcrumbs, parsley, thyme, half the lemon zest, the garlic, a tiny amount of salt (remember, the Parmesan is salty) and some pepper.

Brush the pumpkin generously with olive oil and sprinkle with the crust mix, making sure the slices are covered with a nice, thick coating. Gently pat the mix down a little.

Place the pan in the oven and roast for about 30 minutes, or until the pumpkin is tender: stick a little knife in one wedge to make sure it has softened and is cooked through. If the topping starts to darken too much during cooking, cover loosely with foil.

Mix the sour cream with the dill and some salt and pepper. Serve the wedges warm, sprinkled with the remaining lemon zest, with the sour cream on the side.

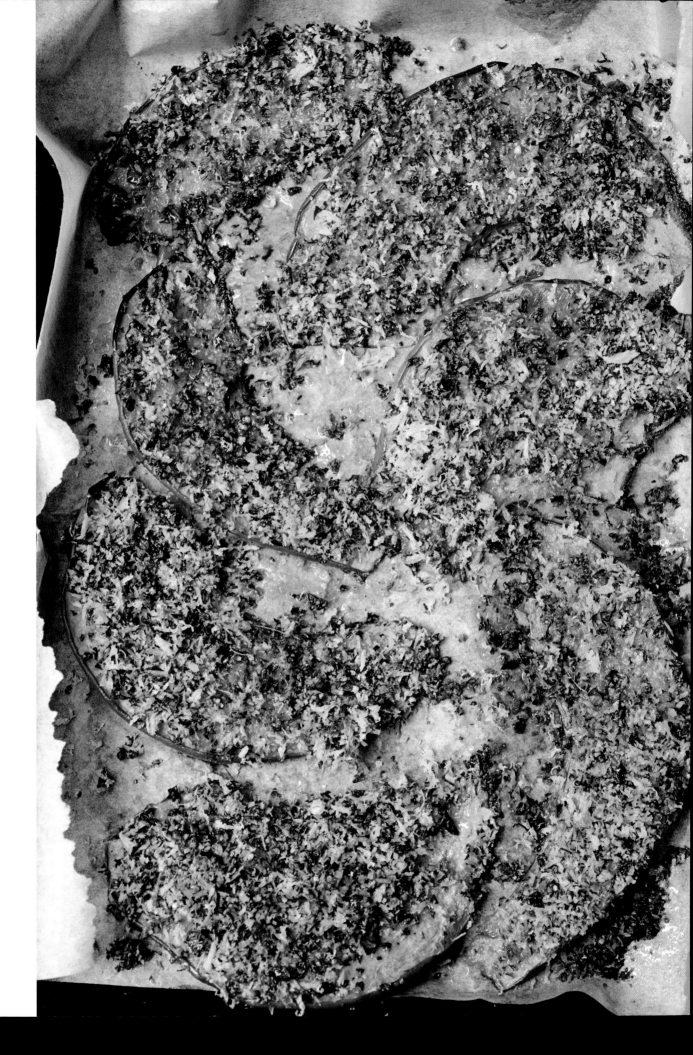

# Tamara's ratatouille

Although I call this ratatouille the name doesn't do it any justice, as this is the most magnificently delicious dish, nothing like the drab pile of limp zucchini I'd normally associate with the name. I was given the recipe by Tamara Meitlis, a friend and a wise cook who would tell you – and I can't agree more here – to get *all* your veg prep done before you start cooking. I also advise you to follow the instructions closely; overcooking the vegetables is exactly the point here.

Serves 4

7 tbsp sunflower oil

2 small onions, cut into 1¼-inch dice

4 garlic cloves, sliced

½ fresh green chile, thinly sliced

2 small red peppers, cut into 1¼-inch dice

½ small butternut squash, peeled and cut into 1¼-inch dice

1 small parsnip, peeled and cut into 1¼-inch dice

1 cup French beans, trimmed

1 medium zucchini, cut into 1¼-inch dice

½ large eggplant, peeled and cut into 1¼-inch dice

1 small potato, peeled and cut into 1¼-inch dice

2 medium tomatoes, peeled and chopped

½ tbsp sugar

1 tbsp tomato paste

salt and black pepper

1 cup water

chopped cilantro to garnish (optional)

Pour two-thirds of the oil into a large heavy casserole dish or a pot and place on a medium–high heat. Add the onions and fry for 5 minutes, stirring occasionally. Next, stir in the garlic, chile and red peppers and fry for another 5 minutes. Add the squash and parsnip and continue frying for 5 minutes.

Using a slotted spoon, lift the vegetables out of the pot and into a medium bowl, leaving as much of the oil in the pot as possible. Top this up with the remaining oil. Add the French beans, zucchini and eggplant to the hot oil and fry for 5 minutes, stirring occasionally.

Return the contents of the bowl to the pot. Add the potato, tomatoes, sugar, tomato paste and plenty of salt and pepper. Stir well, then pour in the water, or just enough to half-cover the vegetables. Cover with a lid and leave to simmer gently for 30 minutes. Taste the vegetables and add more salt and pepper, if you like.

Finally, preheat the oven to 400°F. Use a slotted spoon to gently lift the vegetables from the pot and into a large, deep roasting pan to make a layer about 1¼ inches thick. Pour the liquid over the vegetables and place in the oven to cook for 30 minutes. At this point all the vegetables should be very soft and most of the liquid evaporated. Garnish with cilanro, if you like, and serve.

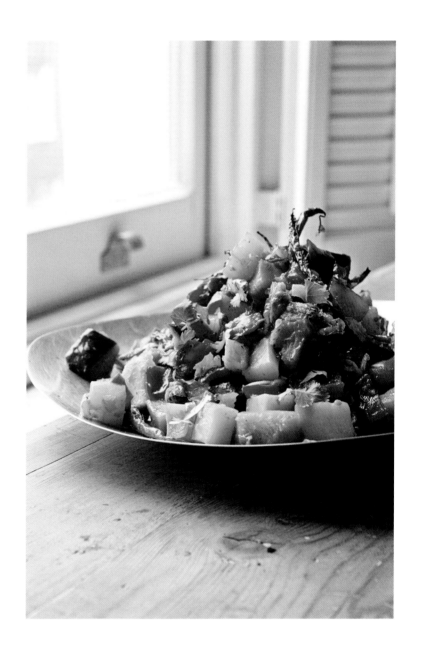

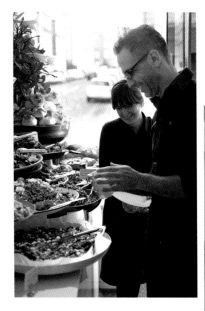

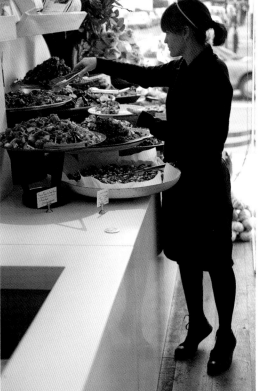

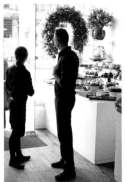

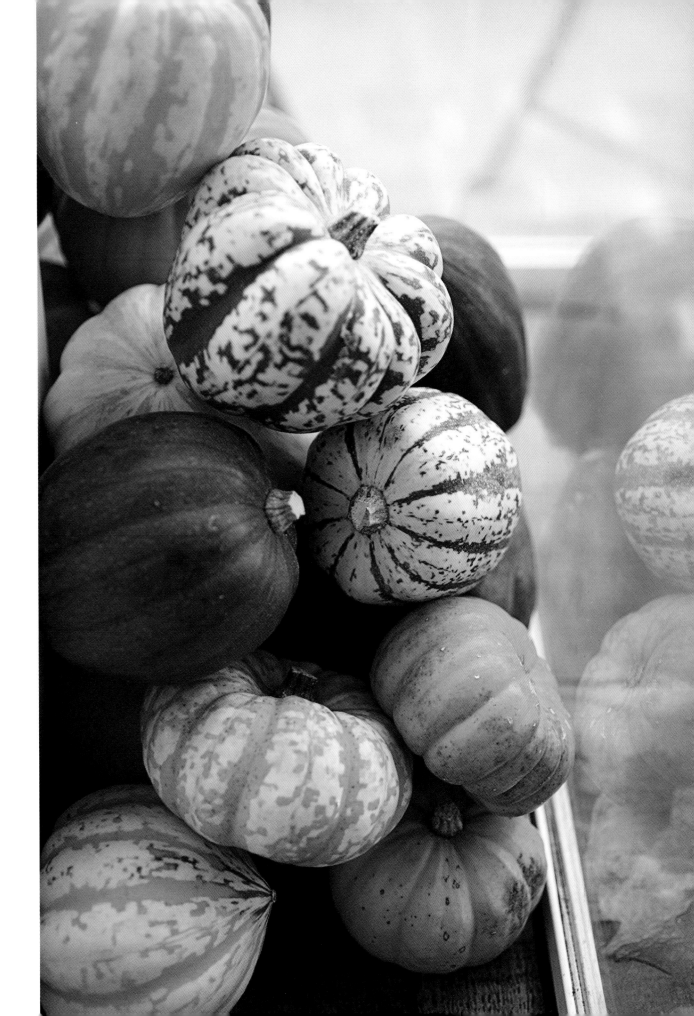

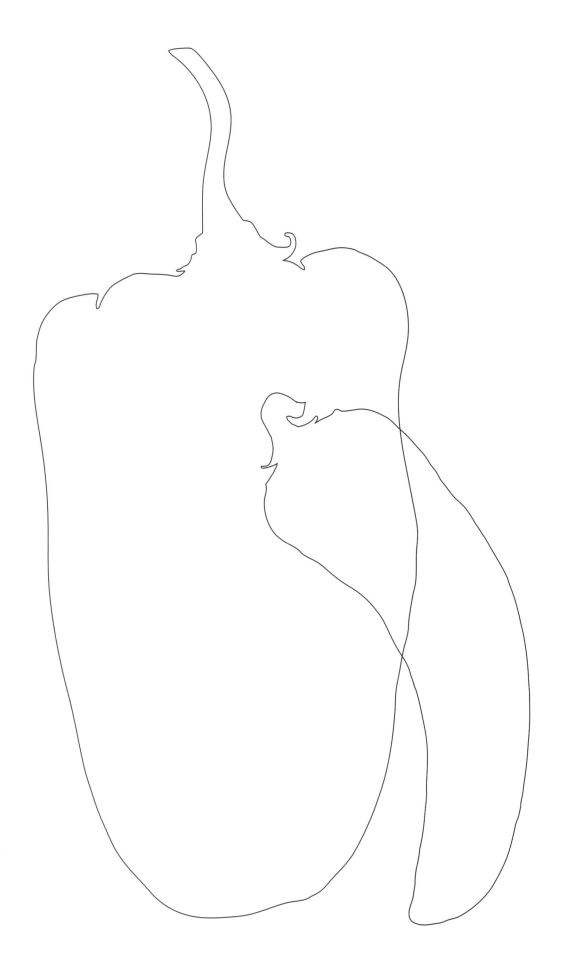

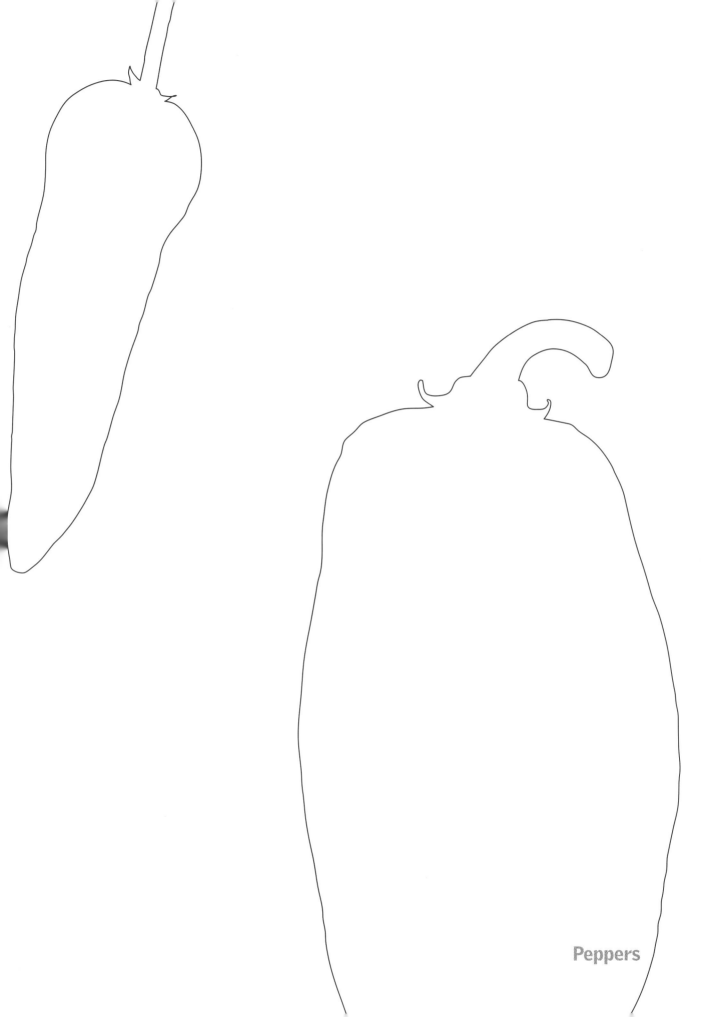

Peppers

# Multi-vegetable paella

All my Spanish ingredients, and lots of other delicious wonders, I get at a small Spanish supermarket, Garcia, on Portobello Road. This is a proper piece of Spain in central London, not only for the produce but also for the typical laid-back attitude. I can't be sure but I think they take a siesta in the middle of the day. Calasparra rice and other good-quality Spanish products can be bought from LaTienda.com in the United States.

Serves 2 generously
3 tbsp olive oil
½ Spanish onion, finely chopped
1 small red bell pepper, cut into strips
1 small yellow bell pepper, cut into strips
½ fennel bulb, cut into strips
2 garlic cloves, crushed
2 bay leaves
¼ tsp smoked paprika
½ tsp ground turmeric
¼ tsp cayenne pepper
1 cup Calasparra rice (or another short-grain paella rice)
6½ tbsp good-quality sherry
1 tsp saffron threads
salt
2 cups boiling vegetable stock
¾ cup shelled fava beans (fresh or frozen)
12 plum tomatoes, halved
5 small grilled artichokes in oil from a jar, drained and quartered
15 pitted kalamata olives, crushed or halved
2 tbsp roughly chopped parsley
4 lemon wedges

Heat up the olive oil in a paella pan, or a large shallow skillet, and gently fry the onion for 5 minutes. Add the bell peppers and fennel and continue to fry on medium heat for about 6 minutes, or until soft and golden. Add the garlic and cook for 1 minute more.

Add the bay leaves, paprika, turmeric and cayenne to the vegetables and stir well. Then add the rice and stir thoroughly for 2 minutes before adding the sherry and saffron. Boil down for a minute, then add the stock and ⅓ teaspoon salt. Reduce the heat to the minimum and simmer very gently for about 20 minutes, or until most of the liquid has been absorbed by the rice. Do not cover the pan and don't stir the rice during the cooking.

Meanwhile, pour plenty of boiling water over the fava beans in a bowl and leave for a minute, then drain well and leave to cool down. Now squeeze each bean gently to remove the skin and discard it.

Remove the paella pan from the heat. Taste and add more salt if needed but without stirring the rice and vegetables much. Scatter the tomatoes, artichokes and fava beans over the rice and cover the pan tightly with foil. Leave to rest for 10 minutes.

Take off the foil. Scatter the olives on top of the paella and sprinkle with parsley. Serve with wedges of lemon.

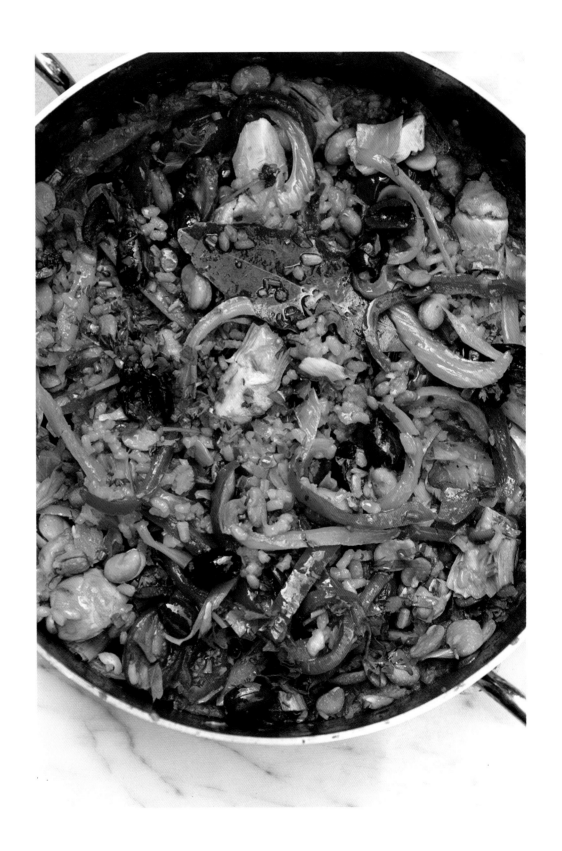

# Marinated pepper salad with pecorino

Crusty bread is essential to soak up the sweet dressing left after finishing this salad. Serve as a starter, followed by a main course of Mushroom and Herb Polenta (page 264).

Serves 2 as a starter
1 red bell pepper, quartered
1 yellow bell pepper, quartered
4 tbsp olive oil
salt
1 tbsp balsamic vinegar
1 tbsp water
½ tsp muscovado sugar
2 thyme sprigs
1 garlic clove, thinly sliced
black pepper
2 tbsp flat-leaf parsley, leaves picked
⅔ cup basil leaves
1 cup watercress
2 oz mature pecorino, shaved
1 tbsp drained capers

Preheat the oven to 375°F. Toss the peppers with 1 tablespoon of the oil and a little salt. Scatter in a roasting pan and roast for 35 minutes, or until they soften and take on some color. Remove to a bowl and cover it with plastic wrap. Once cooled to room temperature, peel the peppers and cut into thick strips.

Whisk together 2 tablespoons of the oil, the balsamic vinegar, water, sugar, thyme, garlic, and some salt and pepper. Pour this over the peppers and leave aside for at least an hour, or overnight in the fridge.

To assemble the salad toss together the herbs, watercress, drained pepper strips, pecorino and capers. Add the remaining 1 tablespoon olive oil and 1 tablespoon (or more if you like) of the marinade. Taste and adjust the seasoning as needed.

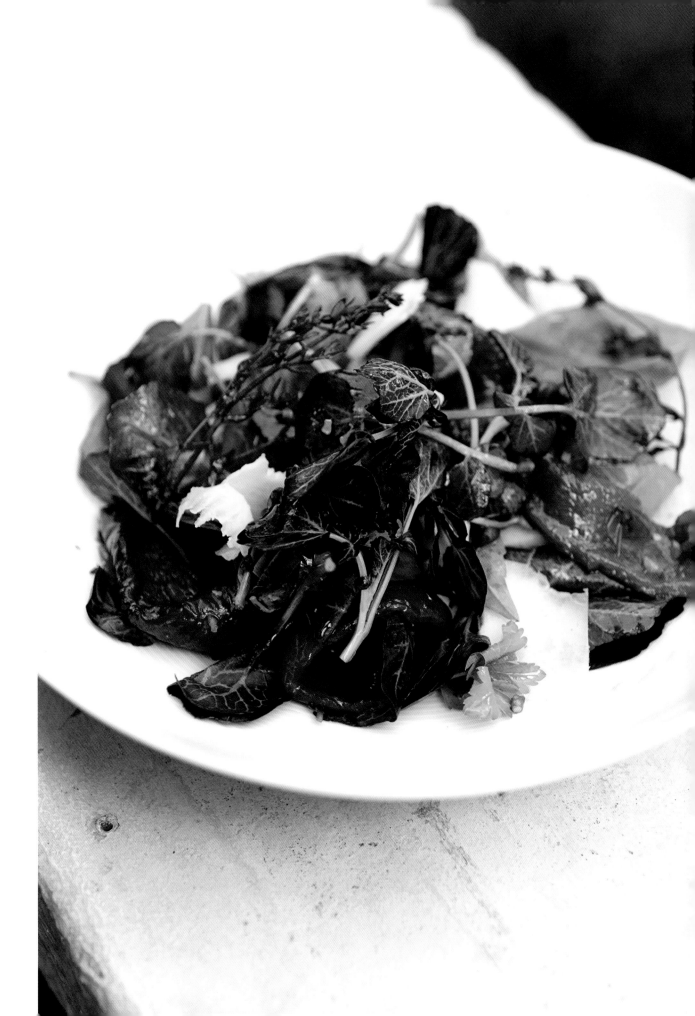

# Very full tart

A fantastic Mediterranean feast, full to the brim with roasted vegetables.

Serves 4–6
1 red bell pepper
1 yellow bell pepper
about 6 tbsp olive oil
1 medium eggplant, cut into 2-inch dice
salt and black pepper
1 small sweet potato, peeled and cut
    into 1-inch dice
1 small zucchini, cut into 1-inch dice
2 medium onions, thinly sliced
2 bay leaves
11 oz pie crust dough
8 thyme sprigs, leaves picked
⅓ cup ricotta
4¼ oz feta
7 cherry tomatoes, halved
2 medium eggs
1 cup heavy cream

Preheat the oven to 450°F. Use a small serrated knife to cut around the stem of the peppers and lift it out along with the seeds. Shake the peppers to remove all the remaining seeds; discard the stems and seeds. Place the two peppers in a small ovenproof dish, drizzle with a little oil and put on the top shelf in the oven.

Mix the eggplant in a bowl with 4 tablespoons of olive oil and some salt and pepper. Spread in a large baking pan and place in the oven on the shelf beneath the peppers.

After 12 minutes add the sweet potato dice to the eggplant pan and stir gently. Return to the oven to roast for another 12 minutes. Then add the zucchini to the pan, stir and roast for a further 10 to 12 minutes. At this point the peppers should be brown and the rest of the vegetables cooked. Remove all from the oven and reduce the temperature to 325°F. Cover the peppers with foil and cool, then peel and tear roughly into strips.

Heat 2 tablespoons of olive oil in a frying pan on medium heat. Sauté the onions with the bay leaves and some salt for 25 minutes, stirring occasionally, until they turn brown, soft and sweet. Remove from the heat, discard the bay leaves and set aside.

Lightly grease a 9-inch loose-bottomed tart pan. Roll out the pie crust dough to a circle roughly ⅛ inch thick and large enough to line the pan, plus extra to hang over the rim. Carefully line the pan with the dough, pressing it into the corners and leaving the excess hanging over the top edge. Line the dough with a large sheet of parchment paper and fill it with pie weights or dried beans. Bake the crust for 30 minutes. Carefully remove the paper with the weights, then bake for 10 to 15 minutes more, or until it turns golden brown. Remove and allow to cool a little.

Scatter the cooked onion over the bottom of the crust and top with the roasted vegetables, arranging them evenly. Scatter half the thyme leaves over. Next, dot the veg with small chunks of both cheeses and then with the tomato halves, cut-side up.

Whisk the eggs and cream in a small bowl with some salt and pepper. Carefully pour this mix into the tart; the top layer of tomatoes and cheese should remain exposed. Scatter the remaining thyme over the top. Place in the oven and bake for 35 to 45 minutes, or until the filling sets and turns golden. Remove and allow to rest for at least 10 minutes before releasing the tart from the pan and serving.

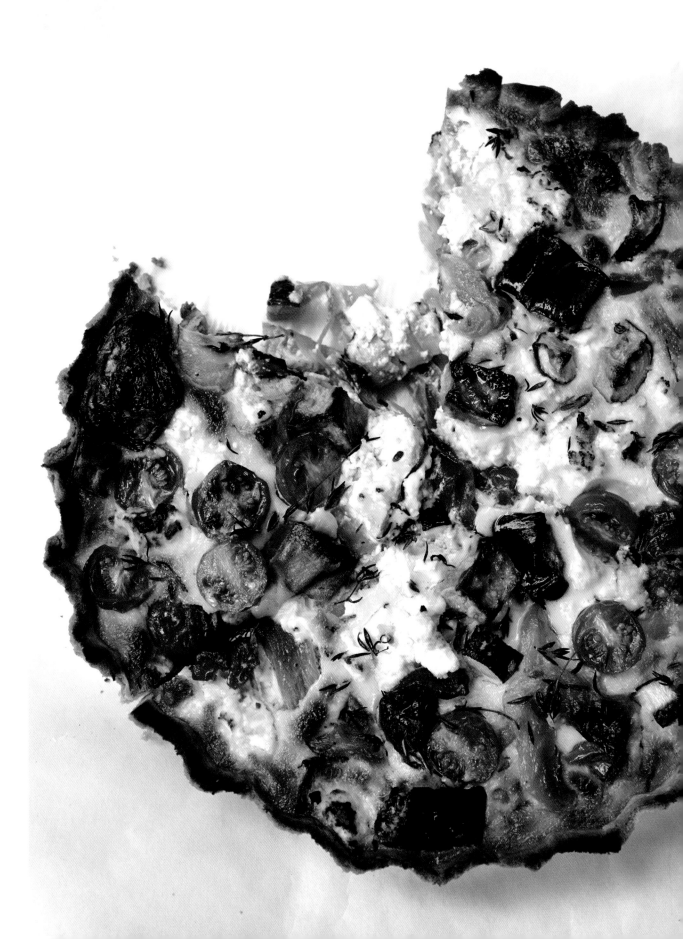

# Scrambled smoky duck eggs on sourdough

This brilliant brunch grub relies on chipotles – smoke-dried jalapeño peppers – which give out a terrific smoky flavor that is warm, earthy and not too spicy. This Mexican staple will add depth and pungency to all stew-type dishes. You can find them at penzeys.com and other online suppliers of chiles.

Serves 4

4 dried chipotle peppers
4 thick slices sourdough bread
lightly salted butter
2 tbsp olive oil
4 garlic cloves, sliced
4 green onions, cut into ¾-inch-long
    pieces
4 plum tomatoes, roughly chopped
6 duck eggs
1 tsp Maldon sea salt
black pepper
bunch of cilantro leaves, roughly
    chopped
4 heaped tbsp sour cream

First, place the dried chipotles in a bowl, cover with boiling water and leave to soak for 15 minutes. Then drain, chop into rough chunks and set aside.

Preheat the grill to high. Place the sourdough bread slices under the grill and toast well on both sides. Spread butter generously on the toasts and leave them somewhere warm.

Heat up the olive oil in a large frying pan. Add the garlic and green onions and cook lightly on medium–high heat. When they begin to turn golden, add the chopped tomatoes and chipotles and cook for a further 1 to 2 minutes.

Break the eggs into a bowl and beat lightly with a fork, adding the salt and some pepper. Pour the eggs into the frying pan and cook for 20 to 30 seconds, stirring constantly to create runny scrambled eggs.

Put the toasts on serving plates, spoon the eggs on top and sprinkle over the cilantro. Serve immediately, with the sour cream on top or on the side.

# Shakshuka

In a tiny alley in old Jaffa there's a little restaurant serving food to customers sitting outside at shared shabby tables. The place is heaving around lunchtime and everybody, more or less, is eating the same thing. The place is called Dr. Shakshuka, after its signature dish, and this is, obviously, what everybody's tucking into.

Shakshuka (pictured on pages 88 to 89) is a North African dish with many variations. Some add preserved lemon, others feta and different herbs and spices. It is my ideal brunch fare! Cook and serve it in individual pans, if you have them, or in one very large one. Chunky white bread on the side is a must.

Serves 4 generously
½ tsp cumin seeds
¾ cup light olive oil or vegetable oil
2 large onions, sliced
2 red bell peppers, cut into ¾-inch strips
2 yellow bell peppers, cut into ¾-inch strips
4 tsp muscovado sugar
2 bay leaves
6 thyme sprigs, leaves picked and chopped
2 tbsp chopped parsley
2 tbsp chopped cilantro, plus extra to garnish
6 ripe tomatoes, roughly chopped
½ tsp saffron threads
pinch of cayenne pepper
salt and black pepper
up to 1⅛ cups water
8 eggs

In a very large pan dry-roast the cumin seeds on high heat for 2 minutes. Add the oil and onions and sauté for 5 minutes. Add the peppers, sugar and herbs and continue cooking on high heat for 5 to 10 minutes to get a nice color.

Add the tomatoes, saffron, cayenne and some salt and pepper. Reduce the heat to low and cook for 15 minutes. During the cooking keep adding water so that the mix has a pasta sauce consistency. Taste and adjust the seasoning. It should be potent and flavorful. (You can prepare this mix well in advance.)

Remove the bay leaves, then divide the pepper mix among four deep frying pans, each large enough to take a generous individual portion. Place them on medium heat to warm up, then make two gaps in the pepper mix in each pan and carefully break an egg into each gap. Sprinkle with salt and cover the pans with lids. Cook on a very (!) gentle heat for 10 to 12 minutes, or until the eggs are just set. Sprinkle with cilantro and serve.

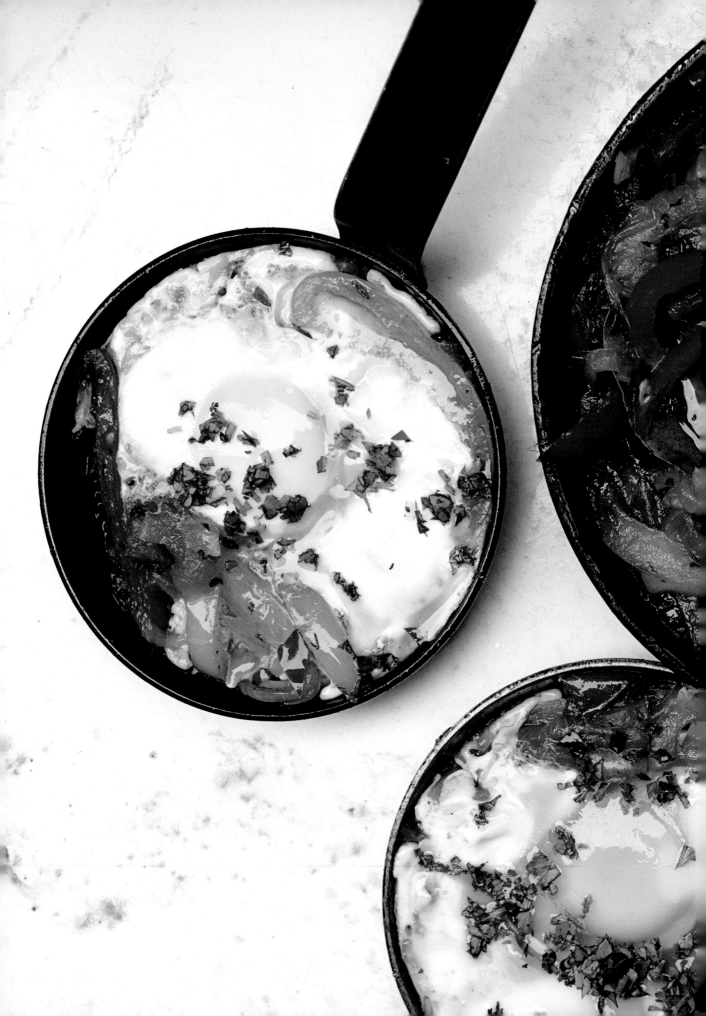

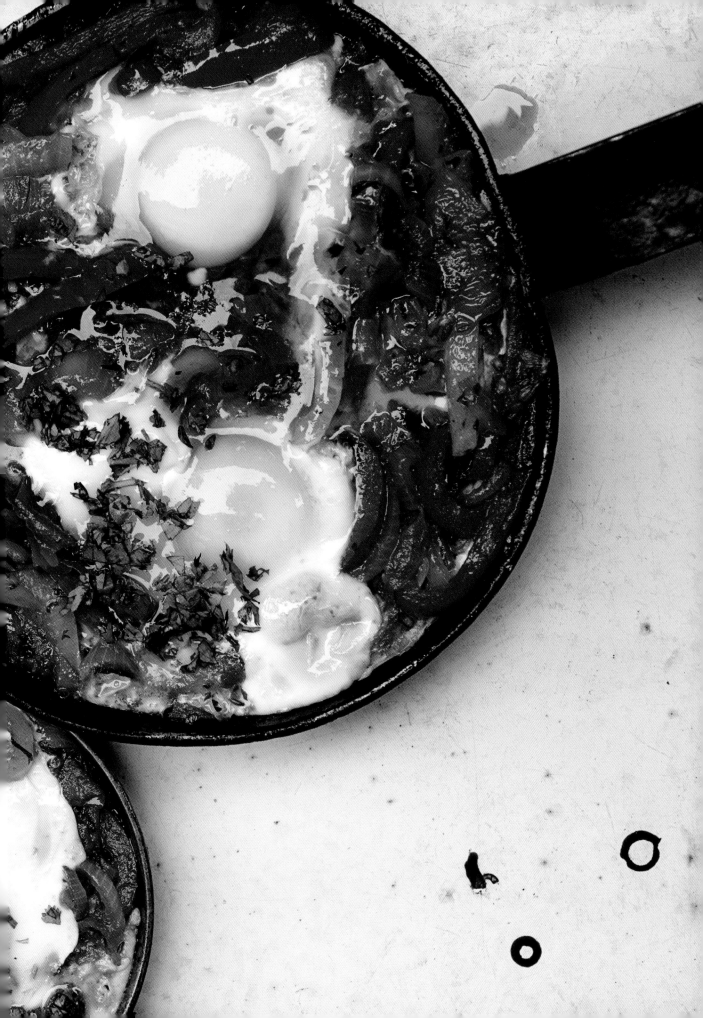

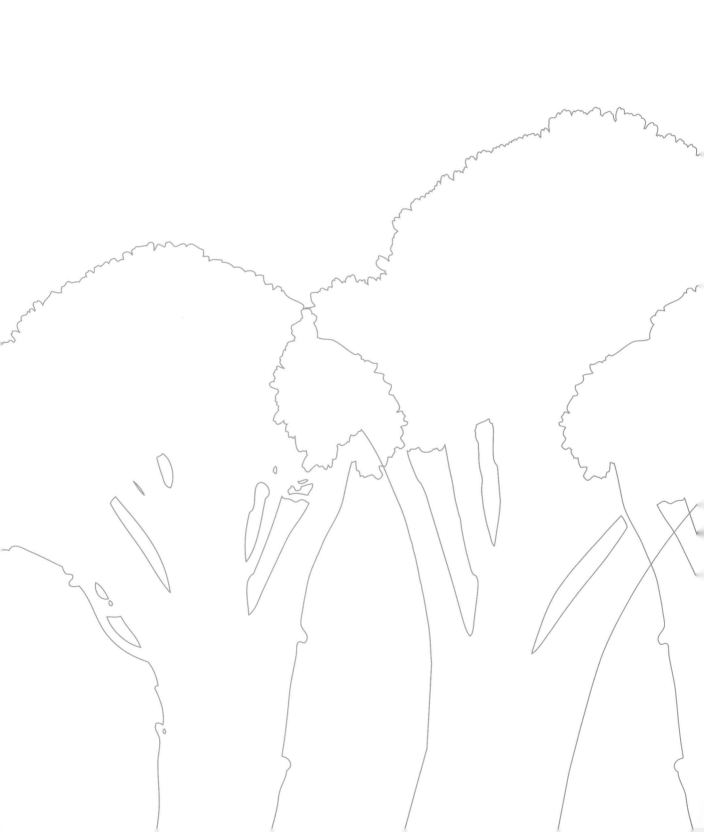

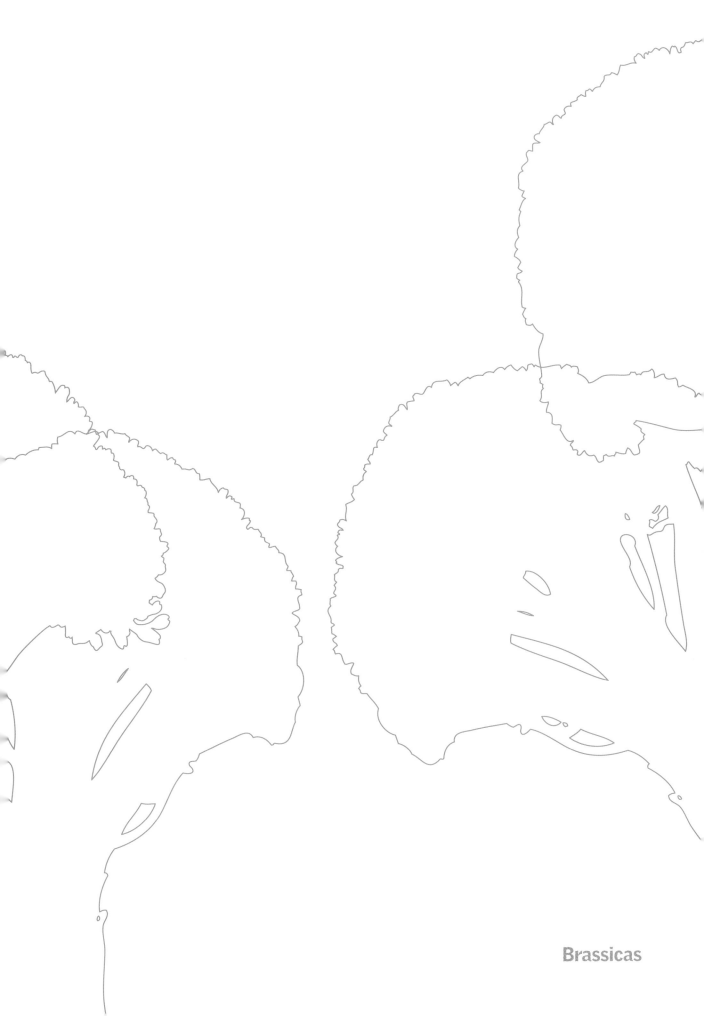

Brassicas

# Broccoli and Gorgonzola pie

Soon after I published this recipe, an annoyed *Guardian* reader sent a letter grumbling about the amount of fat in the pie. His comment somehow managed to unsettle my normally-very-good-tempered self. I guess it was the moralistic tone of the reproach, a condescending attempt by someone who, I suspect, doesn't really like food to tell others what to eat.

I say, enjoy this pie fully! I suggest serving it warm or at room temperature with a simple salad of tomato and red onion, lightly dressed with garlic, olive oil and white wine vinegar.

Serves 6
1 lb puff pastry
2 broccoli heads (1½ lbs in total), cut
    into florets
2 tbsp butter
3 to 4 leeks, trimmed and thinly sliced
⅔ cup heavy cream
⅓ cup water
⅓ cup chopped chives
⅓ cup chopped tarragon
3 tbsp grainy mustard
1 tsp salt
black pepper
7 oz Gorgonzola, cut into medium chunks
1 egg, beaten

Preheat the oven to 400°F. Roll out two-thirds of the pastry into a circle that is ⅛ inch thick and large enough to line a 10-inch loose-bottomed tart pan. Line the pan and trim off the excess pastry. Roll out the remaining pastry into a thinner disc, large enough to cover the surface of the pie, and lay it on a plate. Place both shell and lid in the freezer for 10 minutes.

Line the pastry with parchment paper and fill it with baking beans. Bake blind for 15 to 20 minutes, or until light brown. Remove the paper and beans and return to the oven to bake for about 5 minutes, or until the bottom of the shell is golden. Leave to cool down.

While the tart shell is baking, prepare the filling. Cook the broccoli florets in a large pan of boiling water for about 2 minutes, or until tender but still firm. Drain in a colander, rinse well with cold water and leave to dry.

Melt the butter in a pan and fry the leeks on gentle heat for 10 to 15 minutes, or until soft but not colored. Add the cream, water, chives, tarragon, mustard, salt and some black pepper. Stir well and remove from the heat.

To assemble, spread the leek mixture over the bottom of the pastry case. Scatter the broccoli on top and gently press into the leek mix. Dot with the Gorgonzola. Brush the rim of the tart case with the beaten egg and place the pastry lid over the filling. Press down firmly around the edge to attach the lid to the case. Trim off any of the lid that hangs over the edge.

Glaze the lid with beaten egg and bake for about 30 minutes, or until the pastry is golden brown. Allow to cool a little before removing from the pan.

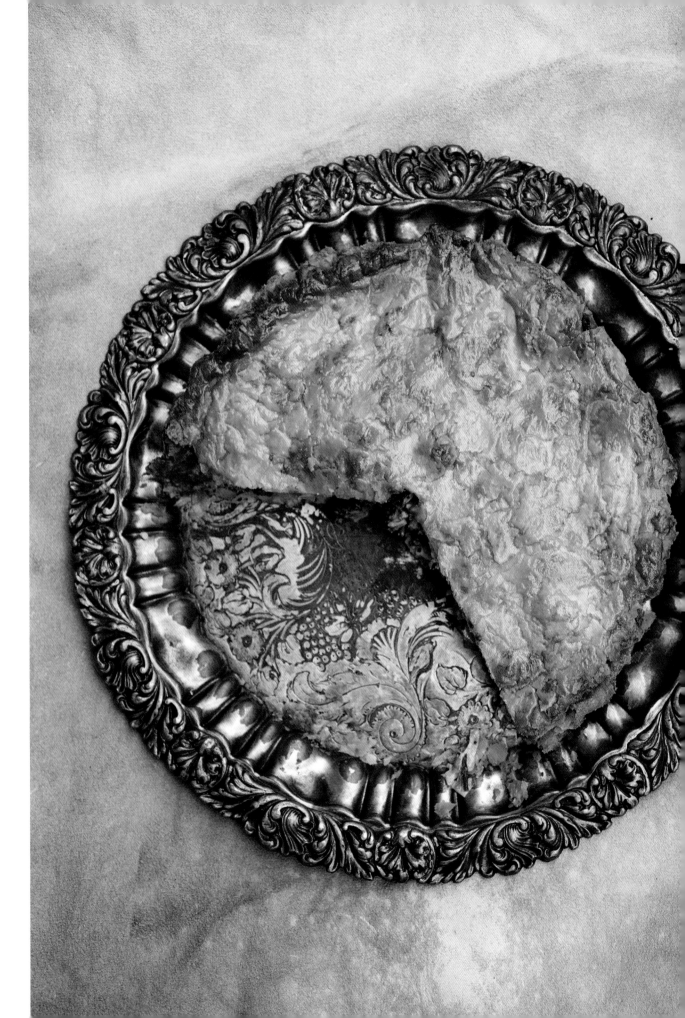

# Broccolini and sweet sesame salad

*Ingen no goma-ae*, Japanese green beans with ground sesame and miso, is a true delicacy. I particularly like it when black sesame seeds are used; they give it an extra-luxurious look. The Japanese dish is the inspiration for this salad, although I must admit the use of tahini is a move no Japanese would ever dream of making. Served with the Quinoa Salad with Dried Persian Lime on page 245 this dish would make a wonderful supper.

Serves 4

Sauce

4 tbsp tahini

2½ tbsp water

1 small garlic clove, crushed

½ tsp tamari

½ tbsp honey

¾ tbsp cider vinegar

1½ tbsp mirin

pinch of salt

¾ lb (3½ cups) broccolini or purple sprouting broccoli

¾ cup green beans

2 cups snow peas

1 tbsp peanut oil

1½ cups cilantro leaves

3 tbsp toasted sesame seeds

1 tsp nigella seeds

To make the sauce. Whisk together all the ingredients in a bowl (reduce the amount of honey if you don't like it too rich). The sauce should be smooth and thick but with a pourable consistency, so adjust the amount of water as necessary. Taste and add more salt, if you like.

Trim off any leaves from the broccolini. If the stalks are thick cut them lengthways into two or four, so you are left with long and thinner stalks, similar in size to the green beans. Trim off the stalk ends of the beans and snow peas, keeping them separate.

Bring a medium pan of unsalted water to the boil. Blanch the green beans for 3 to 5 minutes, or until just tender but still crunchy. Lift into a colander and refresh under running cold water; drain and dry well with a tea towel. In the same water blanch the snow peas for 2 minutes; refresh, drain and dry. Repeat the process with the broccoli, blanching it for 2 to 3 minutes.

Mix all the vegetables together in a bowl with the oil. You can now serve the salad in two ways. For one, stir most of the cilantro leaves and sesame and nigella seeds in with the vegetables and pile up on a serving dish; pour the sauce on top and finish with the remaining cilantro and seeds. Alternatively, pile the vegetables on a serving plate, dotting with cilantro leaves and sprinkling with seeds as you go; serve the sauce in a bowl on the side.

# Stuffed cabbage

This comforting main course makes use of a combination common to Arab and Turkish cuisines – it mixes rice and little vermicelli noodles to create an attractive texture that is light and delicate.

Serves 4

2 tbsp unsalted butter

1½ oz vermicelli noodles (not the rice variety)

⅞ cup basmati rice

1¼ cups water

salt

1 medium white cabbage

⅓ cup pine nuts, toasted and roughly chopped

¾ cup ricotta

¼ cup grated Parmesan

3 tbsp chopped mint

4 tbsp chopped parsley, plus extra to finish

3 garlic cloves, crushed

black pepper

1 cup dry white wine

6 tbsp vegetable stock

1½ tbsp sugar

4 tbsp olive oil

Melt the butter in a small saucepan over a medium heat. Break the vermicelli with your hands into ¾-inch-long pieces and add them to the pan. Stir as you fry them for 1 to 2 minutes. Take care! They can burn in a second. As soon as the noodles start turning golden add the rice and stir well. Then add the water and ½ teaspoon salt and bring to the boil. Turn the heat down to the minimum, cover and cook for 20 minutes. Remove from the heat and leave to sit for 10 minutes before removing the lid and allowing to cool down a bit.

While the rice is cooking, cut the cabbage vertically in half. Peel off the leaves and blanch them in boiling water for 6 to 8 minutes, or until semisoft. You may need to do this in a few batches, depending on the size of your pan. (Alternatively, trim off the base of the cabbage, then put it whole into a pot of boiling water; gradually remove the outer leaves as they cook.) Refresh the leaves under cold running water, drain and pat dry.

Preheat the oven to 350°F. To the cooked rice add the pine nuts, ricotta, half the Parmesan, the herbs, garlic and salt and pepper to taste; mix well with a fork. Use the cooked cabbage leaves to make parcels of whatever size you choose, each one containing a generous amount of the rice filling. Alternatively, make rolls by placing some rice filling at the base of a rectangular-shaped piece of cabbage and then rolling it up; don't worry that the sides remain open.

Arrange the cabbage parcels close together in an ovenproof dish (if you can't fill up the dish completely use cabbage trimmings to fill in the gaps). Whisk together the wine, stock, sugar, olive oil and plenty of salt and pepper. Pour this over the cabbage parcels and put the dish in the oven. Bake for about 40 minutes, or until almost all the liquid is gone. Sprinkle with the remaining Parmesan, return to the oven and bake for a further 10 minutes for the cheese to melt and turn golden. Remove from the oven and allow to rest for 5 minutes before serving.

# Smoky frittata

*Scamorza affumicata* is an Italian cheese that melts fantastically well. Often labelled "smoked mozzarella," it is highly effective in adding depth and pungency to vegetarian dishes.

Serves 4–6
1 small cauliflower, cut into medium
    florets
6 eggs
4 tbsp crème fraîche
2 tbsp Dijon mustard
2 tsp sweet smoked paprika
3 tbsp finely chopped chives
5 oz smoked scamorza, grated
    (including the skin for extra flavor)
2 oz mature Cheddar, grated
salt and black pepper
2 tbsp olive oil

Simmer the cauliflower in a large pan of boiling salted water for only 4 to 5 minutes, or until semi-cooked. Drain and dry.

Preheat the oven to 375°F. Break the eggs into a large bowl. Add the crème fraîche, mustard and paprika and whisk well, making sure the eggs and crème fraîche are thoroughly blended. Now stir in the chives and three-quarters of the cheeses, and season well with salt and pepper.

Heat up the olive oil in a large ovenproof frying pan. Fry the cauliflower for about 5 minutes, or until golden brown on one side. Pour over the egg mixture and use a fork to spread the cauliflower evenly in the pan. Cook on medium heat for about 5 minutes.

Scatter the remaining cheeses on top, then carefully transfer the pan to the oven. Cook for 10 to 12 minutes, or until the frittata is set.

Remove from the oven and let rest for 2 to 3 minutes before cutting into wedges. Eat immediately, with a peppery green salad.

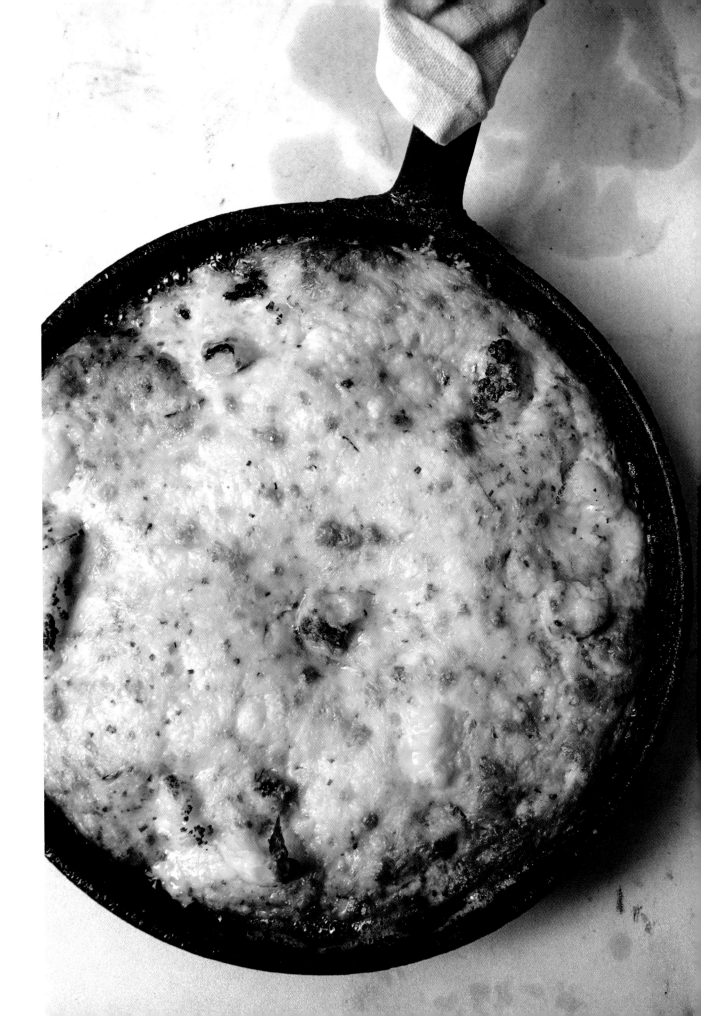

# Purple sprouting broccoli with rice noodles

Yes, there's a long list of ingredients here, but I am ready to be extra-kind and allow you to adapt the recipe, to use commercial Thai curry paste instead of having to schlep and get all the individual items. This "dry" variation of a green curry makes one of the most satisfying supper dishes for the late winter and early months of spring.

Serves 6

Spice paste

¾-inch piece of galangal (or fresh ginger), peeled and chopped

1½ medium fresh green chiles, seeded and roughly chopped

1½ lemongrass stalks, outer layer and tough ends removed, roughly chopped

1 garlic clove, crushed

½ shallot, roughly chopped

¾ tbsp coriander seeds, finely ground

½ tsp cumin seeds, finely ground

grated zest and juice of ½ lime

1 small bunch of cilantro (with stalks and roots)

2 tbsp vegetable oil

1¼ lbs purple sprouting broccoli or broccolini

1 red onion, finely chopped

1 tbsp vegetable oil

salt

1 tsp palm sugar

7 kaffir lime leaves

1¾ cups coconut milk

1 lb wide rice noodles (or rice sticks)

4 tbsp toasted sesame oil

3 tbsp lime juice, plus extra to finish

2 tbsp shredded basil or cilantro

To make the spice paste. Place all the ingredients in the small bowl of a food processor and blend to a paste. You might need to stop once or twice to scrape the mixture back down from the sides of the bowl or add a little extra lime juice or oil. Keep the paste on the side.

Trim any leaves from the broccoli and divide into large florets.

Sauté the onion with the oil in a medium saucepan for 2 to 3 minutes, or until translucent. Add the spice paste and cook, stirring, for 2 minutes. Add 1 teaspoon salt, the palm sugar, lime leaves and coconut milk. Bring to the boil, then turn down the heat and simmer gently for 5 minutes.

Bring two medium saucepans of salted water to the boil. In one, cook the rice noodles for 3 to 6 minutes (check the instructions on the packet) and in the other cook the broccoli for 1 to 2 minutes. Drain both. Rinse the noodles briefly under hot water and drain well, then toss with 3 tablespoons of the sesame oil and the lime juice; season generously with salt. Drizzle the rest of the sesame oil over the broccoli and sprinkle with a pinch of salt.

Divide the noodles among warmed wide bowls and top with the warm broccoli. Spoon 3 to 4 tablespoons of the sauce per portion over and around the broccoli, and finish with the basil or cilantro and a squirt of lime juice.

# Cabbage and kohlrabi salad

People always ask me what to do with kohlrabi, an often unwanted child in the organic vegetable box. It seems too healthful, too weird, too German! In actual fact, this is a wonderful vegetable. When mixed with root vegetables you can use it in gratins; you can shallow-fry it in olive oil and serve with garlic and chives; and you can add it to an Asian stir-fry.

But in this salad (pictured on pages 100 to 101) I think I have found the absolute best use for a kohlrabi. It is wonderfully fresh-tasting, with a good lemony kick and some sharp sweetness. You may end up going looking for kohlrabi, and it isn't very easy to find. Serve the salad alongside rich main courses, such as Very Full Tart (page 84).

Serves 4
1 medium or ½ large kohlrabi
½ white cabbage (8 to 9 oz)
large bunch of dill, roughly chopped
    (6 heaped tbsp)
1 cup dried whole sour cherries
grated zest of 1 lemon
6 tbsp lemon juice
¼ cup olive oil
1 garlic clove, crushed
salt and white pepper
2 cups alfalfa sprouts

Peel the kohlrabi and cut into thick matchsticks that are about ¼ inch wide and 2 inches long. Cut the cabbage into ¼-inch-thick strips.

Put all the ingredients, apart from the alfalfa sprouts, in a large mixing bowl. Use your hands to massage everything together for about a minute so the flavors mix and the lemon can soften the cabbage and cherries. Let the salad sit for about 10 minutes.

Add most of the alfalfa sprouts and mix well again with your hands. Taste and adjust the seasoning; you need a fair amount of salt to counteract the lemon.

Use your hands again to lift the salad out of the mixing bowl and into a serving bowl, leaving most of the juices behind. Garnish with the remaining sprouts and serve at once.

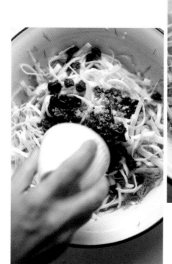
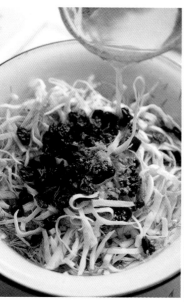
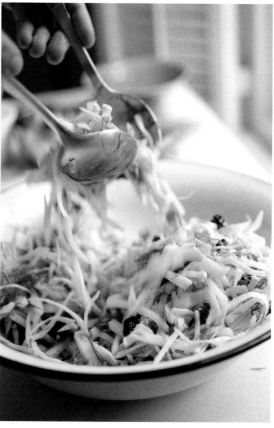

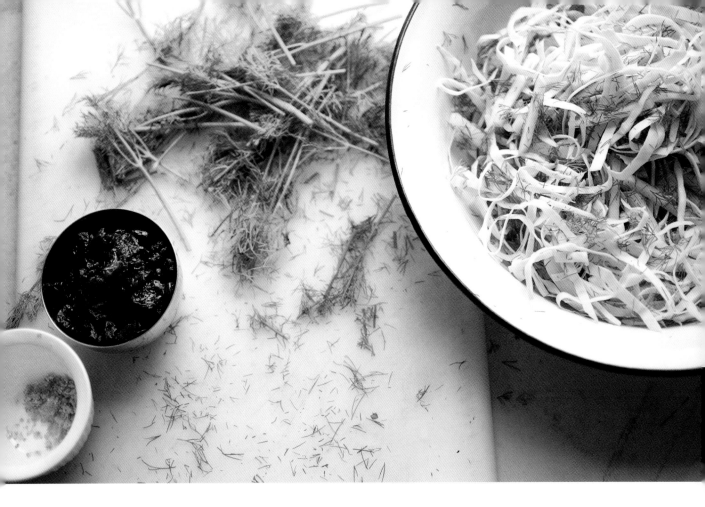

# Sweet winter slaw

This salad will bring color to your winter dinner table and liven up any meal. You can leave out the caramelized macadamias, if you like, or use roasted peanuts instead. Consider serving the slaw with Chard Cakes (page 149) or roast chicken.

Serves 6

**Dressing**

6½ tbsp lime juice

1 lemongrass stalk, chopped into small pieces

3 tbsp maple syrup

2 tbsp toasted sesame oil

1 tsp soy sauce

¼ tsp chile flakes

4 tbsp light olive oil or sunflower oil

1¼ cups macadamia nuts

2 tsp butter

2 tbsp sugar

½ tsp salt

½ tsp chile flakes

7 inner leaves of Savoy cabbage (6 oz in total), finely shredded

½ red cabbage (10 oz), finely shredded

1 mango, cut into thin strips

1 papaya, cut into strips

1 fresh red chile, seeded and finely sliced

¼ cup mint, leaves picked and roughly chopped

1½ cups cilantro, leaves picked and roughly chopped

To make the dressing. Place all the ingredients, except the oil, in a small saucepan and reduce over high heat for 5 to 10 minutes, or until thick and syrupy. Remove from the heat. Once cooled down, strain the sauce into a bowl and add the oil. Put aside for later.

Place the macadamias in a frying pan over medium heat and dry-roast for a few minutes, stirring occasionally, until they are lightly colored on all sides. Add the butter. When it has melted add the sugar, salt and chile flakes. Use a wooden spoon to stir constantly to coat the nuts in the sugar as it caramelizes. Watch carefully as it will only take 1 to 2 minutes and the sugar can burn quickly. Turn out onto a sheet of parchment paper. Cool the nuts, then roughly chop them.

Place the shredded cabbages in a large mixing bowl with the rest of the salad ingredients, including the nuts. Add the dressing and toss together. Taste and add more salt if you need to, then serve.

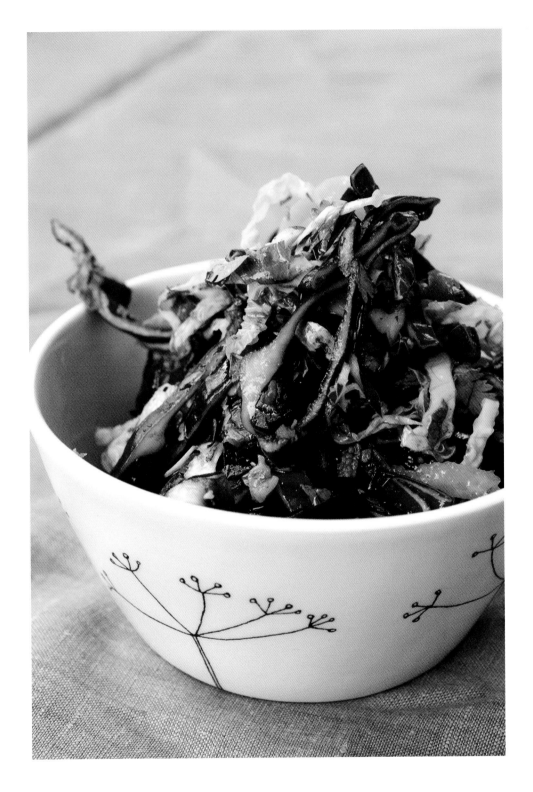

# Savoy cabbage and Parmesan rind soup

This recipe is a bit of a solution – what to do with all the Parmesan rinds left after grating. In restaurants you get loads, so it's common to use them for soups and sauces. At home, you can collect the skins over time and keep them in the freezer. If you don't have enough you can always add more grated Parmesan.

Serves 4

6 tbsp olive oil

1 large onion, sliced

1 garlic clove, crushed

½ tsp caraway seeds, plus extra to garnish

1 medium savoy cabbage

1 medium potato, peeled and diced

5 cups vegetable stock

3 oz Parmesan rinds, plus about ⅓ cup grated Parmesan (optional)

coarse sea salt

½ mild fresh red chile, seeded and thinly sliced

Heat 4 tablespoons of the oil in a large pan and sauté the onion on medium heat for about 5 minutes, or until soft but without much color. Add the garlic and caraway seeds and cook for a further 2 minutes.

Remove four of the outer leaves from the cabbage, shred them finely and put aside for later. Shred the rest of the cabbage leaves roughly and add them to the onions together with the potato. Continue frying, stirring regularly, for 2 to 3 minutes.

Add enough stock just to cover the vegetables and bring to the boil. Add the Parmesan rind, then reduce the heat and simmer for about 10 minutes, or until the potato is tender. Remove and discard the Parmesan rind. Taste the soup and season with salt.

Remove the saucepan from the heat and allow the soup to cool down for a few minutes. Then, using an immersion blender or a regular blender, blitz the soup roughly. Add more stock if you think it is too thick. Adjust the seasoning. Keep hot.

Heat up the remaining 2 tablespoons of oil in a frying pan and sauté the reserved shredded cabbage with the chile and a bit of salt for 3 to 4 minutes, or until the cabbage softens but still retains its vibrant green.

Ladle the hot soup into serving bowls. Add the optional grated Parmesan. Top generously with shredded cabbage and finish with a few caraway seeds.

# Brussels sprouts and tofu

Though unorthodox, here's probably one of the best things you can do with the old Brussels. The delicious sweet sauce lends vibrancy to the dish and makes it utterly addictive. Serve with hot steamed rice.

Serves 4

2 tbsp sweet chile sauce

1½ tbsp soy sauce

3 tbsp toasted sesame oil

1 tsp rice vinegar

1 tbsp maple syrup

5 oz firm tofu

1 lb Brussels sprouts

about ¾ cup sunflower oil

salt

1 cup sliced green onions

½ small fresh red chile, deseeded and finely chopped

1½ cups shiitake mushrooms, halved or quartered

1 cup cilantro leaves

1 tbsp toasted sesame seeds (optional)

Whisk together in a bowl the chile and soy sauces, 2 tablespoons of the sesame oil, the vinegar and maple syrup. Cut the tofu block into ⅜-inch-thick slices and then each slice into two squarish pieces. Gently stir into the marinade and set aside.

Trim the bases off the sprouts and cut each from top to bottom into three thick slices. Take a large nonstick pan, add 4 tablespoons of the sunflower oil and heat up well. Throw in half the sprouts with a little salt and cook on high heat for about 2 minutes. Don't stir much. You want the sprouts to almost burn in a few places and cook through but remain crunchy. Remove to a bowl. Repeat with more oil, salt and the rest of the sprouts. Remove all the sprouts from the pan.

Add 2 more tablespoons of sunflower oil to the pan, heat up and sauté the green onions, chile and mushrooms for 1 to 2 minutes. Transfer to the sprouts bowl.

Leave the pan on high heat. Use tongs to lift half of the tofu pieces from the marinade and gently lay them in the pan (be careful as the oil will spit!), spacing them apart and in one layer. Reduce the flame to medium and cook for 2 minutes on each side, or until they get a nice caramelized color. Transfer to the sprout bowl and repeat with the rest of the tofu.

Once all the tofu is cooked, remove the pan from the heat and return all the cooked ingredients to it. Add the remaining tofu marinade and half the cilantro leaves. Toss everything together and allow to cool down slightly in the pan. Taste and add salt, if needed. Stir in the remaining sesame oil (plus extra, if you like). Serve warm, but not hot, garnished with the sesame seeds, if using, and the rest of the cilantro.

# Saffron cauliflower

In the summer of 2009 I was asked by the makers of the *Food Programme* on BBC Radio 4 to host a half-hour show on a subject of my choice. Bizarrely, I ended up doing a program about cauliflower, trying to show how this veg is unjustifiably losing its popularity in recent years, particularly to broccoli. I know that there's nothing obviously sexy about cauliflower to warrant star status. In fact, it seems – on the face of it – somehow dull and dreary. But as we were working on the show I realized that this isn't really the case, that cauliflower is actually wonderfully versatile, much more so than broccoli. Both Sami Tamimi, Ottolenghi's executive head chef, and I agreed that it is one of those singular vegetables, like potato or eggplant, that can take on big flavors without losing its own unique character.

Here's one example. Serve it as part of a mezze selection or as a side dish with lentils or fish. To upgrade, drizzle with tahini sauce.

Serves 4 as a side dish

1½ tsp saffron

⅓ cup boiling water

1 medium cauliflower, divided into medium florets

1 large red onion, sliced

⅔ cup golden raisins (if they are very dry soak them in water for a few minutes, then drain)

½ cup good-quality green olives, pitted and cut lengthways in half

4 tbsp olive oil

2 bay leaves

salt and black pepper

4 tbsp roughly chopped parsley

Preheat the oven to 400°F. Put the saffron strands in a small bowl and pour over the boiling water. Leave to infuse for a minute, then pour the saffron and water into a large mixing bowl. Add the remaining ingredients, except the parsley, and mix everything together well with your hands.

Transfer the mix to a medium ovenproof dish, cover with foil and place in the oven. Cook for 40 to 45 minutes, or until the cauliflower is tender but still a bit firm, not soft. Halfway through the cooking time remove the dish from the oven and stir well, then cover again and return to bake.

Once the cauliflower is cooked, take it out of the oven, remove the foil and allow to cool down slightly before stirring in the parsley. Taste and adjust the seasoning, then serve warm or at room temperature.

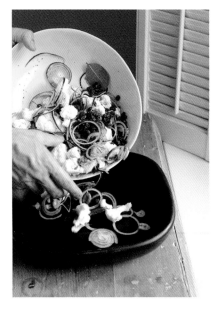
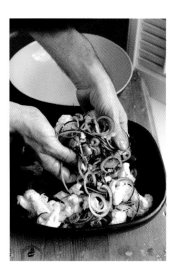

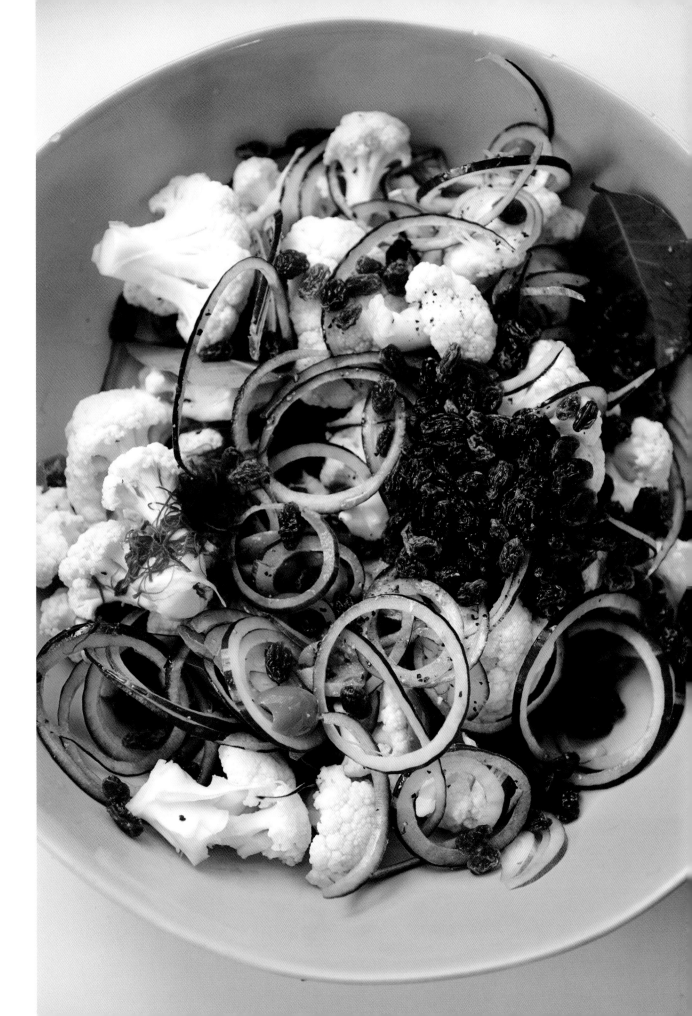

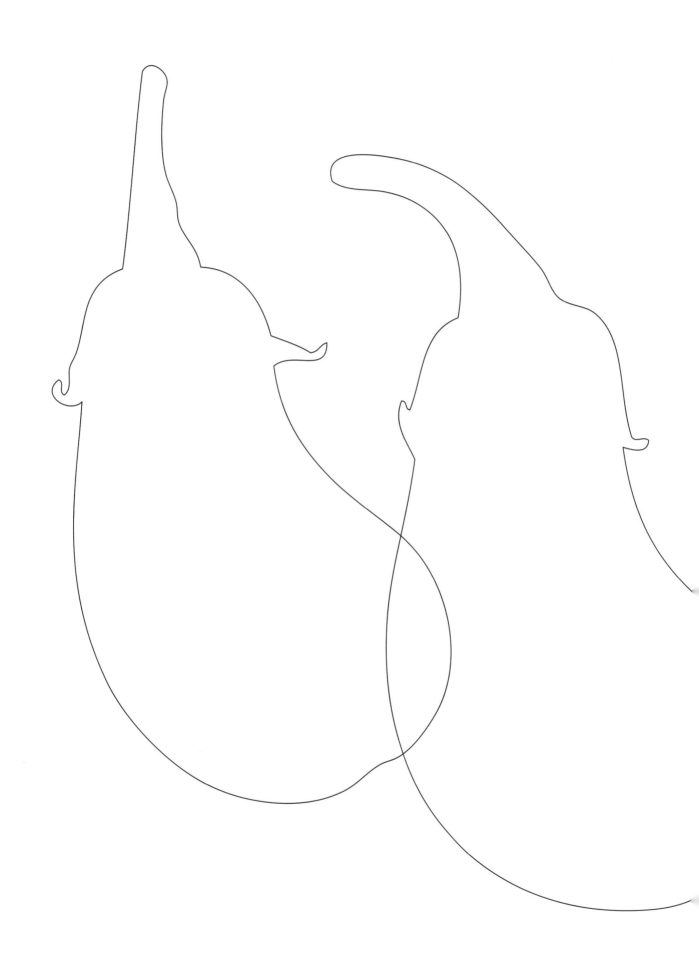

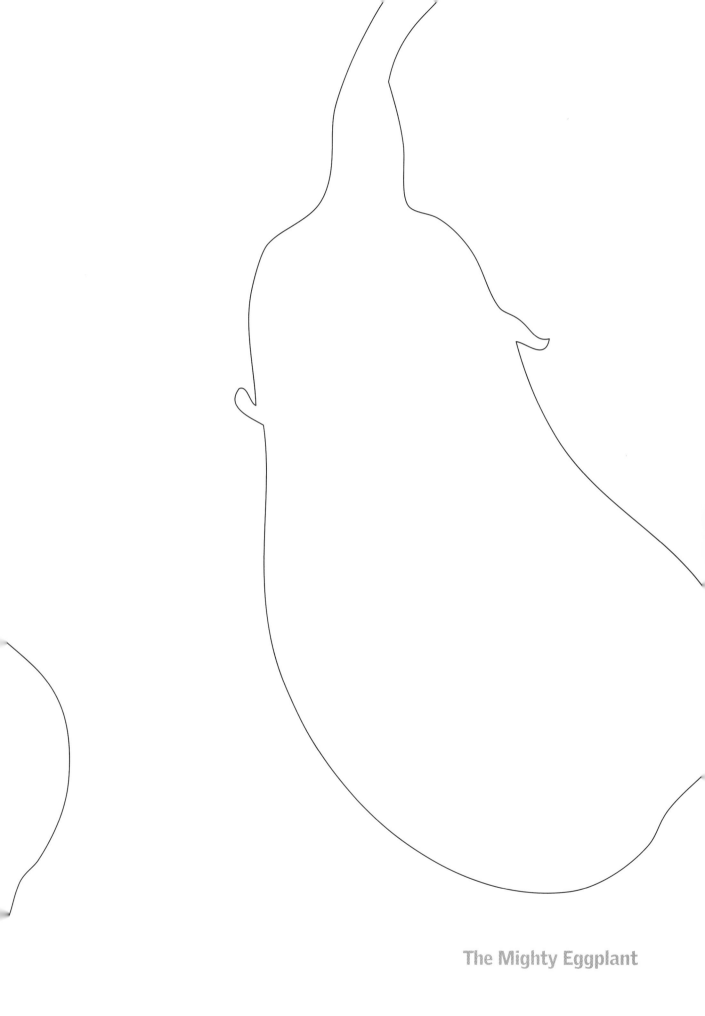

The Mighty Eggplant

# Eggplant with buttermilk sauce

I can't think of a more rustically elegant (is that a contradiction in terms?) starter. Serve with some robust white bread or pita and you are, literally, in food heaven. In the recipe you'll find Sami Tamimi's technique for getting the seeds out of the pomegranate, which I am afraid is now a very well-known secret.

Serves 4 as a starter
2 large and long eggplants
⅓ cup olive oil
1½ tsp lemon thyme leaves, plus a few
    whole sprigs to garnish
Maldon sea salt and black pepper
1 pomegranate
1 tsp za'atar

Sauce
9 tbsp buttermilk
½ cup Greek yogurt
1½ tbsp olive oil, plus a drizzle to finish
1 small garlic clove, crushed
pinch of salt

Preheat the oven to 400°F. Cut the eggplants in half lengthways, cutting straight through the green stalk (the stalk is for the look; don't eat it). Use a small sharp knife to make three or four parallel incisions in the cut side of each eggplant half, without cutting through to the skin. Repeat at a 45-degree angle to get a diamond-shaped pattern.

Place the eggplant halves, cut-side up, on a baking sheet lined with parchment paper. Brush them with olive oil – keep on brushing until all of the oil has been absorbed by the flesh. Sprinkle with the lemon thyme leaves and some salt and pepper. Roast for 35 to 40 minutes, at which point the flesh should be soft, flavorful and nicely browned. Remove from the oven and allow to cool down completely.

While the eggplants are in the oven, cut the pomegranate into two horizontally. Hold one half over a bowl, with the cut side against your palm, and use the back of a wooden spoon or a rolling pin to gently knock on the pomegranate skin. Continue beating with increasing power until the seeds start coming out naturally and falling through your fingers into the bowl. Once all are there, sift through the seeds to remove any bits of white skin or membrane.

To make the sauce. Whisk together all of the ingredients. Taste for seasoning, then keep cold until needed.

To serve, spoon plenty of buttermilk sauce over the eggplant halves without covering the stalks. Sprinkle za'atar and plenty of pomegranate seeds on top and garnish with lemon thyme. Finish with a drizzle of olive oil.

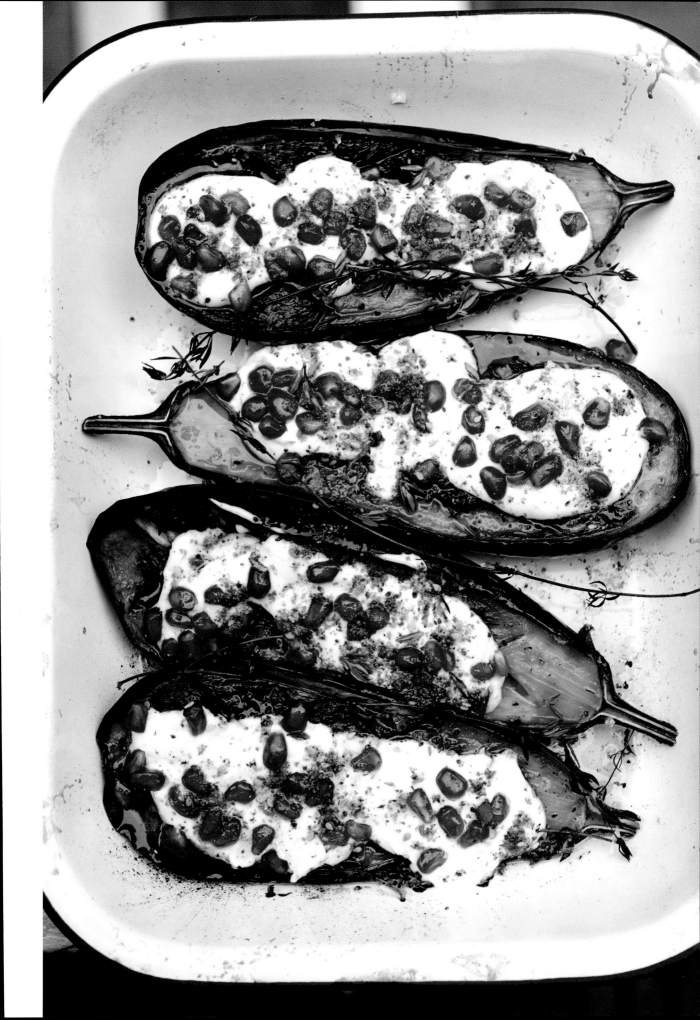

# Soba noodles with eggplant and mango

This dish has become my mother's ultimate cook-to-impress fare. And she is not the only one, as I have been informed by many readers. It is the refreshing nature of the cold buckwheat noodles (see more about them in Soba noodles with wakame, page 188), the sweet sharpness of the dressing and the muskiness of mango that make it so pleasing. Serve this as a substantial starter or turn it into a light main course by adding some fried firm tofu.

Serves 6

½ cup rice vinegar

3 tbsp sugar

½ tsp salt

2 garlic cloves, crushed

½ fresh red chile, finely chopped

1 tsp toasted sesame oil

grated zest and juice of 1 lime

1 cup sunflower oil

2 eggplants, cut into ¾-inch dice

8 to 9 oz soba noodles

1 large ripe mango, cut into ⅜-inch dice or into ¼-inch-thick strips

1⅔ cup basil leaves, chopped (if you can get some use Thai basil, but much less of it)

2½ cups cilantro leaves, chopped

½ red onion, very thinly sliced

In a small saucepan gently warm the vinegar, sugar and salt for up to 1 minute, just until the sugar dissolves. Remove from the heat and add the garlic, chile and sesame oil. Allow to cool, then add the lime zest and juice.

Heat up the sunflower oil in a large pan and shallow-fry the eggplant in three or four batches. Once golden brown remove to a colander, sprinkle liberally with salt and leave there to drain.

Cook the noodles in plenty of boiling salted water, stirring occasionally. They should take 5 to 8 minutes to become tender but still al dente. Drain and rinse well under running cold water. Shake off as much of the excess water as possible, then leave to dry on a dish towel.

In a mixing bowl toss the noodles with the dressing, mango, eggplant, half of the herbs and the onion. You can now leave this aside for 1 to 2 hours. When ready to serve add the rest of the herbs and mix well, then pile on a plate or in a bowl.

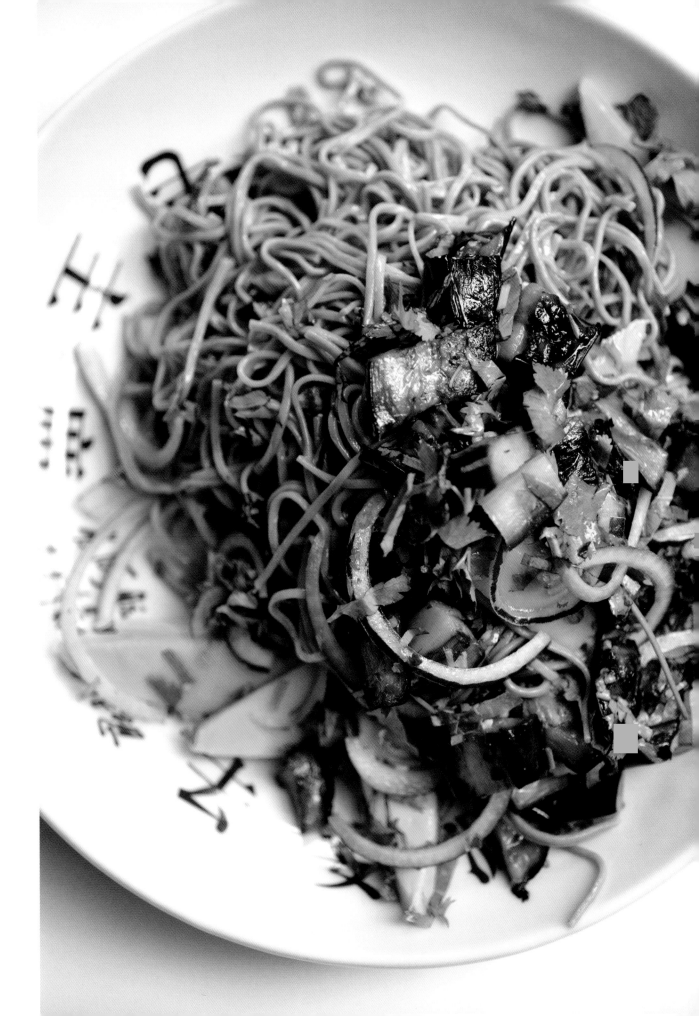

# Eggplant tricolore (and more)

I hope all Italians will be able to forgive me for this – the sacrilegious use of cilantro in a very Italian dish. In fact, and I say so quietly, almost in a whisper, it works marvellously well. And I'd go even further into very dangerous territory by suggesting, God forbid, that fresh cilantro could fit perfectly in traditional Italian cuisine. That's it, I've said it. Now feel free to substitute good old basil for the cilantro.

Serves 4

3 medium eggplants

olive oil

Maldon sea salt and black pepper

1 yellow bell pepper, cut into ⅜-inch dice

10 cherry tomatoes, quartered

1 tbsp red wine vinegar

3½ tbsp capers, plus 1 tbsp of the caper brine

5 oz top-quality buffalo mozzarella

1 cup picked coriander leaves

Preheat the oven to 375°F. Cut the eggplants widthways into ¾-inch-thick slices. Place the slices on a baking sheet lined with parchment paper. Brush them generously on both sides with plenty of oil and sprinkle with salt and pepper. Roast in the oven for 25 to 30 minutes, or until the eggplants are soft and golden brown. Allow to cool down.

Mix together the bell pepper, tomatoes, vinegar, capers and brine, and 2 tablespoons of olive oil. Set aside for at least 30 minutes (the mix can be kept refrigerated for several days; the flavors will deepen over time).

To serve, arrange the eggplant slices, slightly overlapping, on a serving dish. Break the mozzarella into large chunks and scatter on top. Spoon over the yellow pepper salsa and finish with the cilantro.

# Broiled vegetable soup

The process of broiling the vegetables before cooking them together gives this soup a profound depth of flavor. It keeps well so double it and it will sustain you kindly.

Serves 4

3 medium eggplants
2 red bell peppers, stems removed with seeds
3 medium tomatoes
2 red onions, finely diced
2 tbsp olive oil
¾ cup basil leaves, torn
4 oregano sprigs, leaves picked
10 garlic cloves, peeled
1 qt vegetable stock
salt and black pepper
4 cups freshly cooked lima beans (canned are also okay)
4 tbsp Greek yogurt or 4 lemon quarters

Preheat the broiler to high. Line a small baking pan with foil. Prick the eggplants in a few places with a small pointy knife and place in the pan. Broil for 30 minutes.

Place the bell peppers in another small foil-lined baking pan under the broiler, next to the eggplants. Turn the eggplants over with tongs. Broil for 15 minutes, turning the peppers over once during this time. Don't worry if the eggplant skin begins to crack and char or if the peppers start going black.

Place the whole tomatoes in a small pan, underneath the other vegetables. Continue broiling the vegetables for 15 minutes. Then remove them all from the broiler. Cover the peppers with foil and leave to cool down; once they can be handled, peel them and tear the flesh into pieces. Cut a long slit in each eggplant and scoop out the soft flesh, avoiding most of the burnt skin; roughly chop the flesh and set aside.

While the vegetables are broiling, put the onions and olive oil in a large pot and fry on low heat for about 20 minutes, or until the onions are soft and golden.

Add the eggplant flesh, peppers, tomatoes, half the basil, the oregano leaves, garlic, stock and some salt and pepper. Bring to the boil, then simmer the soup for 15 minutes.

Blitz until smooth using an immersion blender, or a regular blender. Add the beans and mix well. Reheat the soup, then taste for seasoning. Serve hot, topped with a dollop of Greek yogurt (or with lemon) and the remaining basil.

# Lentils with broiled eggplant

A most delicious main course for any occasion, formal or casual. After the recipe appeared in the *Guardian* I received two anxious letters from readers who had experienced mini-explosions in their kitchen. Apparently – and I didn't know it then – in some cases eggplants under the broiler can explode with a thunderous boom, the flesh spouting everywhere, rather than deflate gradually as the skin burns and breaks. I sincerely apologize to all who had this experience. So please make sure to pierce the eggplants!

Serves 4

2 medium eggplants

2 tbsp top-quality red wine vinegar

salt and black pepper

1 cup small dark lentils (such as Puy or Castelluccio), rinsed

3 small carrots, peeled

2 celery stalks

1 bay leaf

3 thyme sprigs

½ white onion

3 tbsp olive oil, plus extra to finish

12 cherry tomatoes, halved

⅓ tsp brown sugar

1 tbsp each roughly chopped parsley, cilantro and dill

2 tbsp crème fraîche (or natural yogurt, if you prefer)

To cook the eggplants on a gas stovetop, which is the most effective way, start by lining the area around the burners with foil to protect them. Put the eggplants directly on two moderate flames and roast for 12 to 15 minutes, turning frequently with metal tongs, until the flesh is soft and smoky and the skin is burnt all over. Keep an eye on them the whole time so they don't catch fire. For an electric stove, pierce the eggplants with a sharp knife in a few places. Put them on a foil-lined tray and place directly under a hot broiler for 1 hour, turning them a few times. The eggplants need to deflate completely and their skin should burn and break.

Remove the eggplants from the heat. If you used an oven broiler, change the oven to its normal setting. Heat the oven to 275°F. Cut a slit down the center of the eggplants and scoop out the flesh into a colander, avoiding the black skin. Leave to drain for at least 15 minutes and only then season with plenty of salt and pepper and ½ tablespoon of the vinegar.

While the eggplants are broiling, place the lentils in a medium saucepan. Cut one carrot and half a celery stalk into large chunks and throw them in. Add the bay leaf, thyme and onion, cover with plenty of water and bring to the boil. Simmer on a low heat for up to 25 minutes, or until the lentils are tender, skimming away the froth from the surface from time to time. Drain in a sieve. Remove and discard the carrot, celery, bay leaf, thyme and onion and transfer the lentils to a mixing bowl. Add the rest of the vinegar, 2 tablespoons of the olive oil and plenty of salt and pepper; stir and set aside somewhere warm.

Cut the remaining carrot and celery into ⅜-inch dice and mix with the tomatoes, the remaining oil, the sugar and some salt. Spread in an ovenproof dish and cook in the oven for about 20 minutes, or until the carrot is tender but still firm.

Add the cooked vegetables to the warm lentils, followed by the chopped herbs and stir gently. Taste and adjust the seasoning. Spoon the lentils onto serving plates. Pile some eggplant in the center of each portion and top it with a dollop of crème fraîche or yogurt. Finish with a trickle of oil.

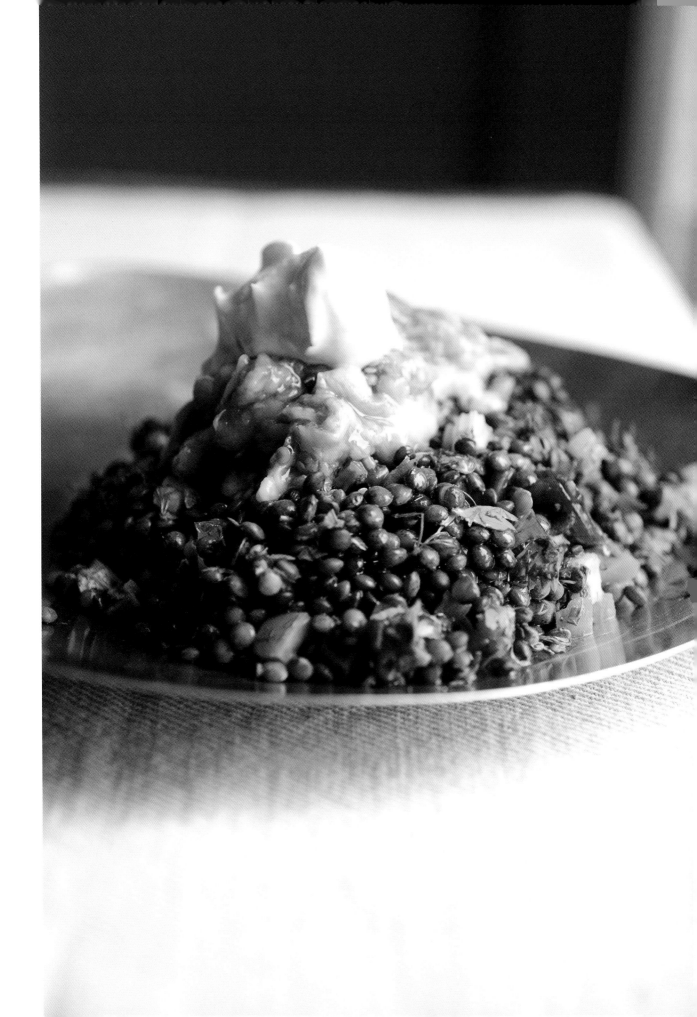

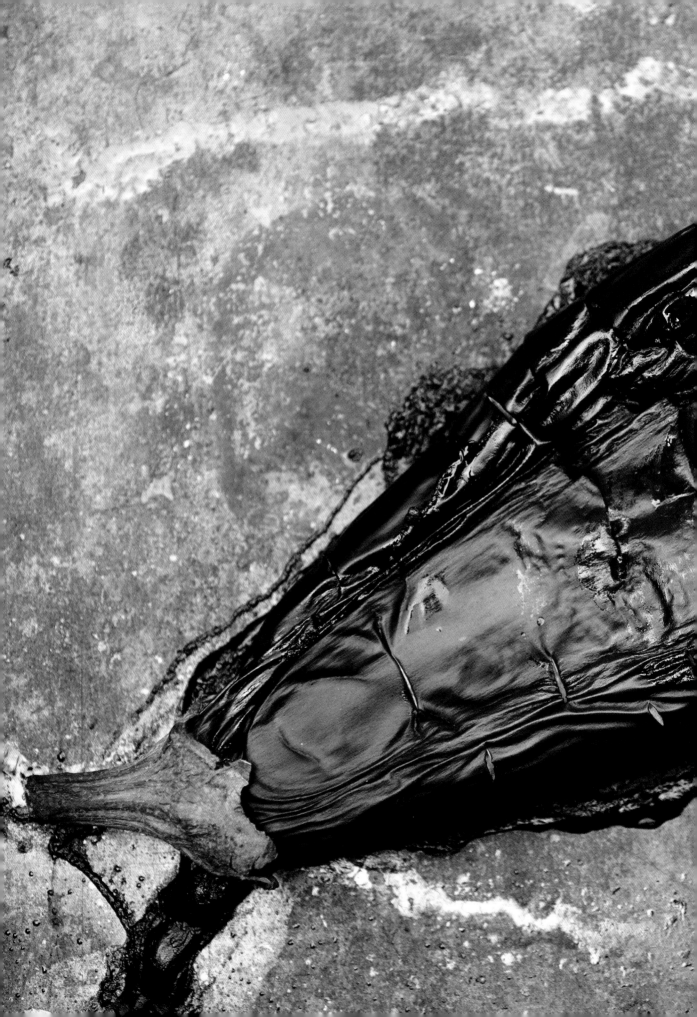

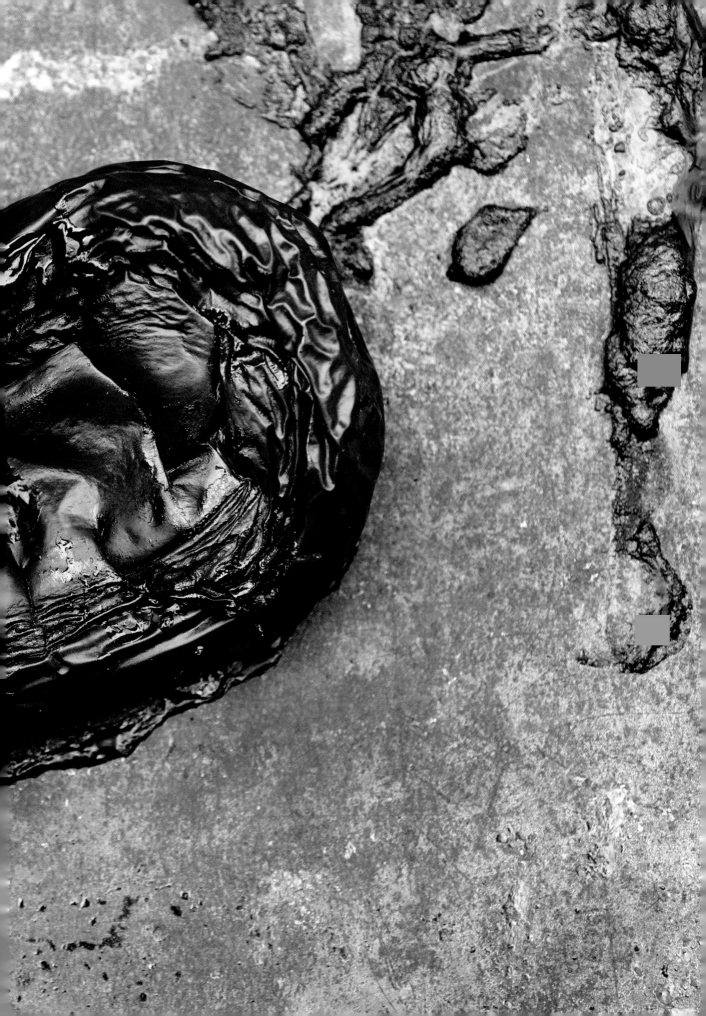

# Eggplant croquettes

My fascination with croquettes started when I was living in Amsterdam, more than a decade ago. As I was often not sober, for all sorts of reasons, I managed to fall in love with a national perversion: warm and cheesy grease balls that came out of a vending machine. I assure you that you'll be able to enjoy my croquettes with a much clearer conscience. Serve them as a nibble or a starter. You can substitute a much simpler wedge of lemon for the aioli, if you prefer.

Serves 6

4 medium eggplants
2 medium russet potatoes, cooked, peeled and smashed
1 large egg, beaten
5 oz feta, crumbled
3 tbsp grated Parmesan
½ tsp salt
black pepper
about 1¾ cups dried white breadcrumbs

Tarragon aioli (optional)

1 egg yolk
1 small garlic clove, crushed
1½ tbsp lemon juice
¼ tsp salt
¼ cup grapeseed oil
¼ cup olive oil
2 tbsp chopped tarragon

sunflower oil for frying

First, burn the eggplants (see page 116). When the eggplants are cool, make a slit along each eggplant and use a spoon to scoop out the flesh; try to avoid the black skin. Place in a colander and discard the rest. Leave to drain for 30 minutes to get rid of some of the liquid. Once drained, you should have roughly 1¼ lbs of eggplant flesh.

Place the eggplant flesh in a large bowl. Add the potatoes, egg, feta, Parmesan, salt and some pepper. Bring everything together gently with a fork; you want to keep the mix quite rough. Add about half of the breadcrumbs, just enough so the mix is sufficiently solid to hold its shape but is still a little sticky.

Remove the mix from the bowl and divide it into four. Roll each portion into a thick sausage that is about 1 inch in diameter. Sprinkle the remaining breadcrumbs on your work surface and roll the sausages in them so they are completely coated. Transfer to a tray and leave to firm up in the fridge for at least 20 minutes.

To make the aioli. Place the egg yolk, garlic, lemon juice and salt in a food processor. Turn the machine on and add the oils, one after the other, in a slow, steady stream. When the aioli is creamy and thick like mayonnaise, fold in the tarragon. Keep in the fridge.

To cook the croquettes, cut each sausage into 2¼-inch-long barrel-shaped pieces; you should end up with about 20 pieces. Pour enough frying oil into a frying pan to come about ¾ inch up the sides. Heat up the oil, then fry the croquettes in small batches for about 3 minutes, turning them over to color evenly. Make sure the oil is always hot but not so hot that it burns the croquettes. Transfer to paper towels to drain. Serve hot.

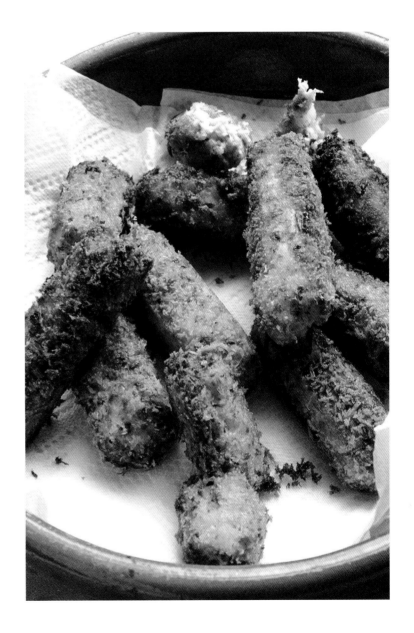

# Burnt eggplant with tahini

This can be a potent dip or condiment that you can serve with raw vegetables or to accompany lamb or fish. Or, with the optional chunks of cucumber and tomato, it can be a gloriously refreshing summer salad that exudes Middle Eastern aromas. You choose.

Serves 2–4
1 large eggplant
⅓ cup tahini paste
¼ cup water
2 tsp pomegranate molasses
1 tbsp lemon juice
1 garlic clove, crushed
3 tbsp chopped parsley
salt and black pepper
3 mini cucumbers (6 to 7 oz in total, optional)
¾ cup cherry tomatoes (optional)
seeds from ½ large pomegranate (see page 110)
a little olive oil to finish

First, burn the eggplant (see page 116). When cool enough to handle scoop out the flesh into a colander, avoiding the blackened skin. Leave to drain for at least 30 minutes.

Chop the eggplant flesh roughly and transfer to a medium mixing bowl. Add the tahini, water, pomegranate molasses, lemon juice, garlic, parsley and some salt and pepper; mix well with a whisk. Taste and adjust the seasoning, adding more garlic, lemon juice or molasses if needed. You want the salad to have a robust sour/ slightly sweet flavor.

If you want to add cucumber and tomatoes, cut the cucumbers lengthways in half and then each half lengthways in two. Cut each quarter into ⅜-inch-long pieces. Halve the tomatoes. Stir them and the cucumber into the eggplant mix.

To serve, spread over a shallow dish, scatter the pomegranate seeds on top and drizzle with oil.

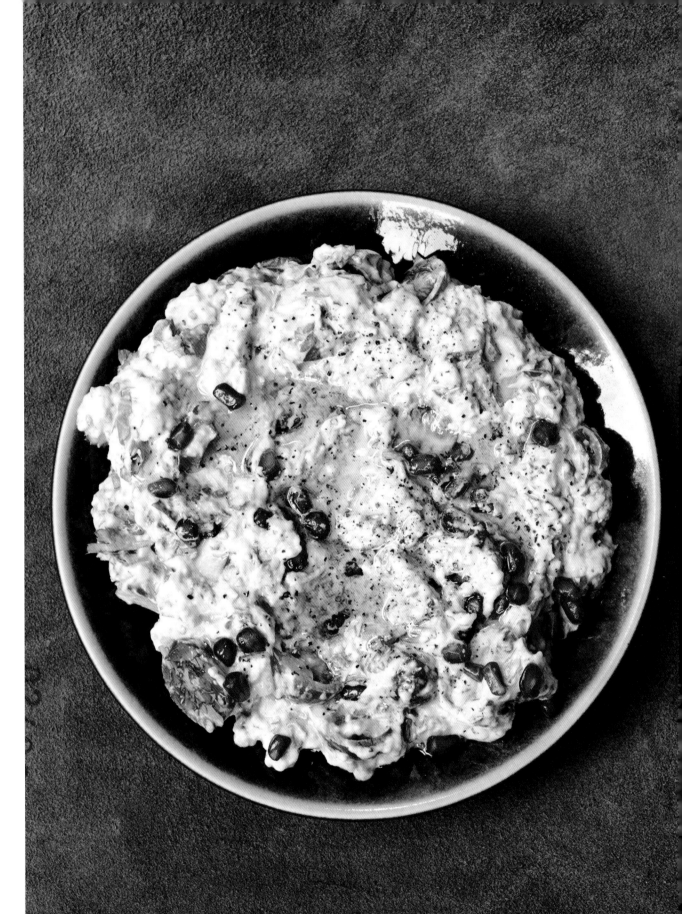

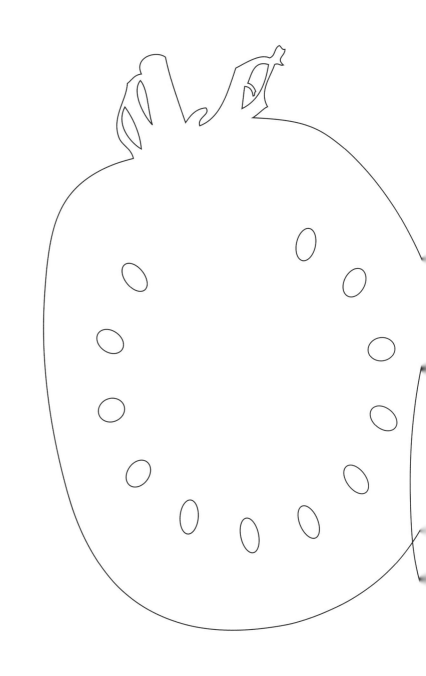

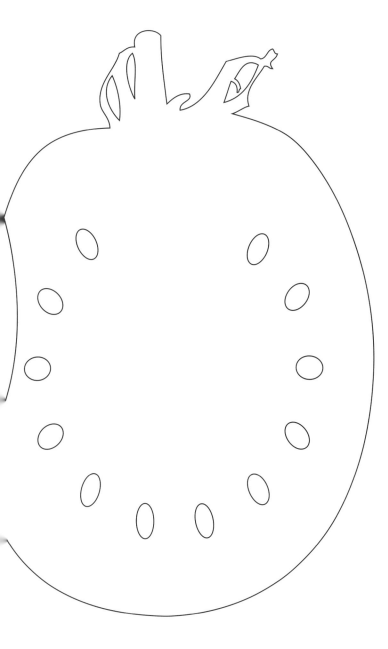

Tomatoes

# Marinated buffalo mozzarella and tomato

This is probably one of the simplest yet finest starters you can offer. There's only one catch – your ingredients. I would ditch the idea at once if I couldn't get a ripe summery tomato, juicy and sweetly intense, a tomato that has never seen a fridge or a chilled truck, only soil and sun. You can actually get such tomatoes if you look hard enough. The best tomato I ever had was homegrown in the village of Monarola in the Cinque Terre, northern Italy. I'll never forget it. You also need a top-quality buffalo mozzarella. Serve this with good crusty white bread.

Serves 4 as a starter

Marinade

½ tsp fennel seeds

grated zest of 1 lemon

15 basil leaves, shredded

2 tsp chopped oregano

2 tsp best-quality extra virgin olive oil,
    plus extra to finish

2 tsp grapeseed oil

1 garlic clove, crushed

½ tsp Maldon sea salt

black pepper

8 to 9 oz buffalo mozzarella

2 ripe medium tomatoes (red, yellow
    or mixed)

To make the marinade. Scatter the fennel seeds in a small frying pan over medium heat and dry-roast until they begin to pop. Transfer to a mortar and pestle and crush roughly. Place the crushed seeds in a small bowl and add the remaining marinade ingredients.

Break the mozzarella roughly with your hands. Smear it with the marinade and set aside for 15 to 30 minutes.

To serve, cut the tomatoes into wedges and plate along with the marinated mozzarella. Drizzle with extra olive oil and serve.

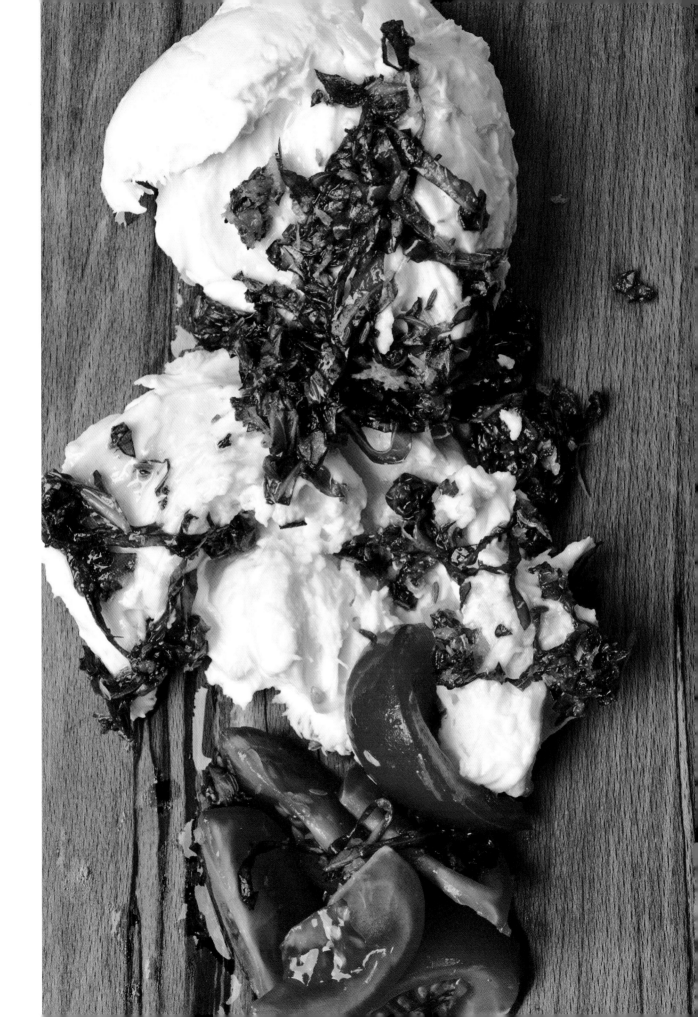

# Quinoa and grilled sourdough salad

This summery bread salad isn't much short of a whole meal. I have taken the traditional Arab fattoush, changed the bread and bulked it up with quinoa, which is the only grain I dare to use in this salad as it's very light and delicate. A lot rests here on the poor tomato. If your tomatoes are sweet and juicy you may not need as much dressing to perk them up. If they are "dry" and bland you may want to add a bit more. Leave the prepared salad to sit a little so the bread croutons can soften up – unless you want them mega-crunchy.

Serves 4

¼ cup quinoa

4 slices sourdough bread

⅓ cup olive oil, plus extra to brush the bread

salt

4 ripe medium tomatoes

3 small cucumbers, unpeeled

½ small red onion, very thinly sliced

4 tbsp chopped cilantro

1½ tbsp chopped mint

2 tbsp chopped parsley

1 tbsp lemon juice

¾ tbsp red wine vinegar

2 small garlic cloves, crushed

black pepper

Preheat the oven to 350°F. Place the quinoa in a saucepan of boiling water and cook for 9 minutes, or until tender. Drain in a fine sieve, rinse under cold water and leave to dry.

Brush the bread with a little bit of olive oil and sprinkle with some salt. Lay the slices on a baking sheet and bake for about 10 minutes, turning them over halfway through. The bread should be completely dry and crisp. Remove from the oven and allow to cool down, then break by hand into different-sized pieces.

Cut the tomatoes into roughly ¾-inch dice and put in a mixing bowl. Cut the cucumbers into similar-size pieces and add to the tomatoes. Add all the remaining ingredients, including the quinoa and croutons, and stir gently until everything is mixed well together. Taste and adjust the seasoning.

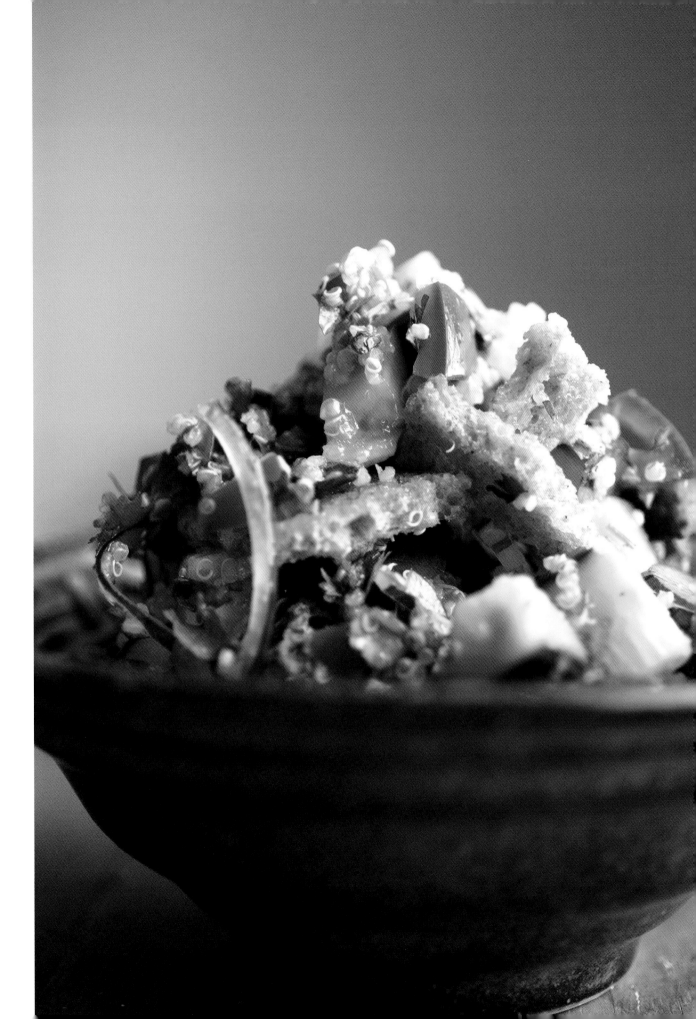

# Tomato, semolina and cilantro soup

Straightforward comfort food at my dad's home was simply cooked semolina with butter and Parmesan. I was looking for a soup containing semolina when I came across a recipe by the famous Israeli chef, Rafi Cohen, whose Moroccan grandmother made a semolina-based soup (as did my Italian grandmother). Here's my variation on his theme.

Serves 6

3 tbsp olive oil

1 medium onion, finely chopped

1 celery stalk, roughly chopped

2 tsp ground coriander

2 tsp ground cumin

1½ tsp sweet paprika

2 tsp finely chopped thyme

3½ cups cilantro leaves, roughly chopped

2 tbsp tomato paste

5 medium tomatoes (1 lb in total), peeled and finely chopped

salt and black pepper

about 6½ cups water

1½ tbsp sugar

1 cup semolina

1½ tbsp lemon juice (optional)

3 tbsp Greek yogurt (optional)

Heat up the olive oil in a medium pot. Add the onion, celery, ground coriander, ground cumin, paprika, thyme and half the chopped cilantro. Sauté on medium heat until the onion is golden and soft. Add the tomato paste and stir for a minute. Add the tomatoes and some salt and pepper, and cook for a few more minutes. Add the water and sugar and bring to the boil, then simmer for 20 minutes.

Next, add the semolina to the simmering soup in a slow stream as you whisk vigorously. Keep on cooking for 10 minutes, whisking occasionally to avoid lumps (don't worry if you do get some after all; they will turn into little dumplings with an appealing texture).

Before serving, add more water if the soup is too thick for your liking. Taste and add more salt and pepper and the lemon juice, if needed. Ladle into bowls, spoon yogurt on top, if you like, and garnish with the remaining chopped cilantro.

# Tomato party

The purpose of this salad (pictured on pages 132 to 133) is to make use of as many as possible of the infinite types of tomatoes that are available now. Some I cook a little, others more, and some I leave completely raw, to maximize the "tomatoey" effect with diverse flavors and textures. Choose whatever tomato selection you can get; the one below is just a suggestion.

Instead of the Sardinian fregola (available from kalustyans.com), you can use Arab mograbiah (from Middle Eastern grocers) or Israeli couscous. Or just leave out the fregola and double the quantity of couscous.

Serves 4
¾ cup couscous
salt
olive oil
⅔ cup boiling water
1 cup fregola
3 medium vine-ripened tomatoes, quartered
¾ tsp brown sugar
black pepper
1 tsp balsamic vinegar
1 cup yellow cherry tomatoes, halved
2 tbsp roughly chopped oregano
2 tbsp roughly chopped tarragon
3 tbsp roughly chopped mint
1 garlic clove, crushed
1 small green tomato, cut into thin wedges
¾ cup red cherry tomatoes, halved

Preheat the oven to 325°F. Put the couscous in a bowl with a pinch of salt and a drizzle of oil. Pour over the boiling water, stir and cover the bowl with plastic wrap. Set aside for 12 minutes, then remove the plastic wrap, separate the grains with a fork and leave to cool.

Place the fregola in a pan of boiling salted water and simmer for 18 minutes, or until al dente. Drain in a colander and rinse under cold running water. Leave to dry completely.

Meanwhile, spread the quartered vine tomatoes over half of a large baking pan and sprinkle with the sugar and some salt and pepper. Drizzle the balsamic vinegar and some oil over the top. Place in the oven. After about 20 minutes remove from the oven and increase the temperature to 400°F. On the empty side of the baking pan, spread the yellow tomatoes. Season them with salt and pepper and drizzle over some oil. Return to the oven and roast for 12 minutes. Remove the tomatoes and allow to cool down.

Mix together the couscous and fregola in a large bowl. Add the herbs, garlic, cooked tomatoes with all their juices, the green tomato and cherry tomatoes. Very gently mix together using your hands. Taste for seasoning: you might need to add salt, pepper and some olive oil.

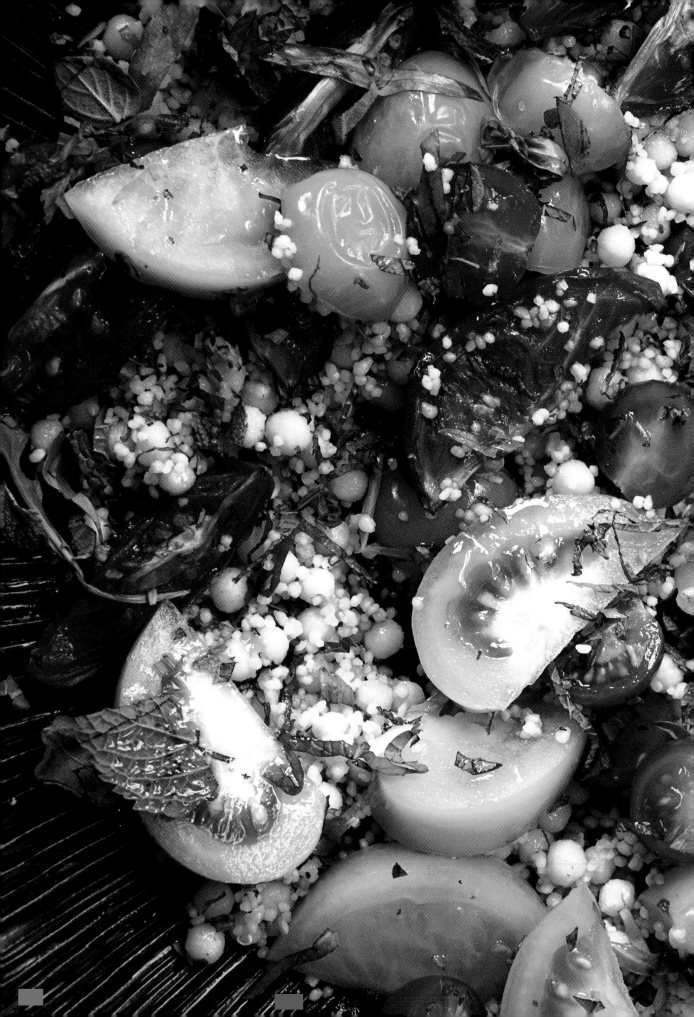

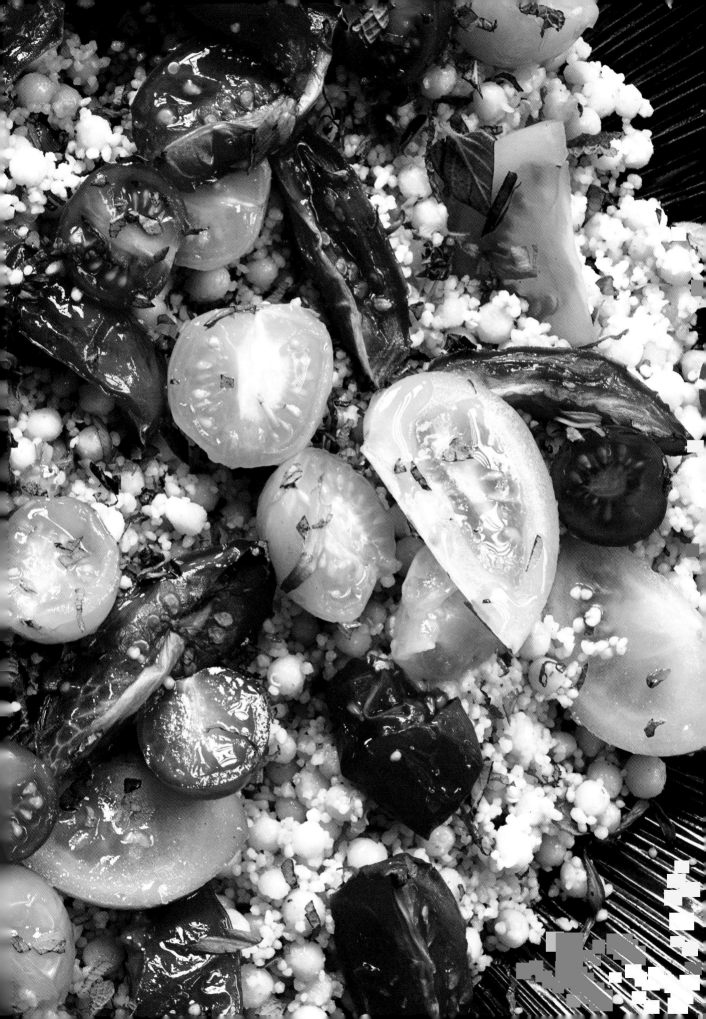

# Quesadillas

While all the meat-eaters are scoffing smoky joints of this, that or the other, try this Mexican sandwich as a vegetarian barbecue dish.

Serves 4

**Black bean paste**

1½ cups cooked black beans (canned are fine)

1 tsp ground coriander

½ tsp ground cumin

¼ tsp cayenne pepper

1 bunch cilantro (leaves and stalks, about 1 oz), chopped

juice of 1 lime

¼ tsp salt

**Salsa**

½ small red onion, thinly sliced

½ tbsp white wine vinegar

3 green onions, thinly sliced

5 medium tomatoes, diced

1 garlic clove, crushed

1 mild fresh red chile, finely diced

1 bunch of cilantro (leaves and stalks, about 1 oz), finely chopped, plus extra leaves to garnish

¾ tsp salt

juice of ½ lime

2 ripe medium avocados, diced

8 small tortillas (preferably corn)

¾ cup sour cream

4½ oz good-quality sharp Cheddar, grated

6 tbsp drained and roughly chopped pickled jalapeños

To make the black bean paste. Place all the ingredients in a food processor and quickly pulse until a rough paste has formed.

Make the salsa. First soak the red onion in the vinegar in a large bowl for a few minutes. Then add all of the other ingredients and stir well.

Prepare the barbecue, or heat a ridged griddle pan.

Take one of the tortillas and spread with 2 tablespoons of the bean paste, creating a large circle in the center but leaving about ¾ inch clear all around at the edge. Over one half of the bean circle spread a tablespoon of sour cream, a sprinkle of Cheddar, a tablespoon of salsa and some jalapeños. Fold over the other tortilla half.

To cook, gently place the quesadillas on the barbecue, or one at a time on the hot griddle pan. Leave for 2 to 3 minutes, then turn and cook for 2 to 3 minutes on the other side. The filling should be warm and the tortilla nicely charred.

Cut each tortilla into two at an angle and transfer to a serving dish. Spoon any remaining salsa alongside and garnish with cilantro leaves.

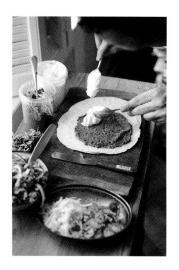
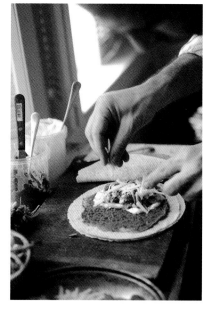

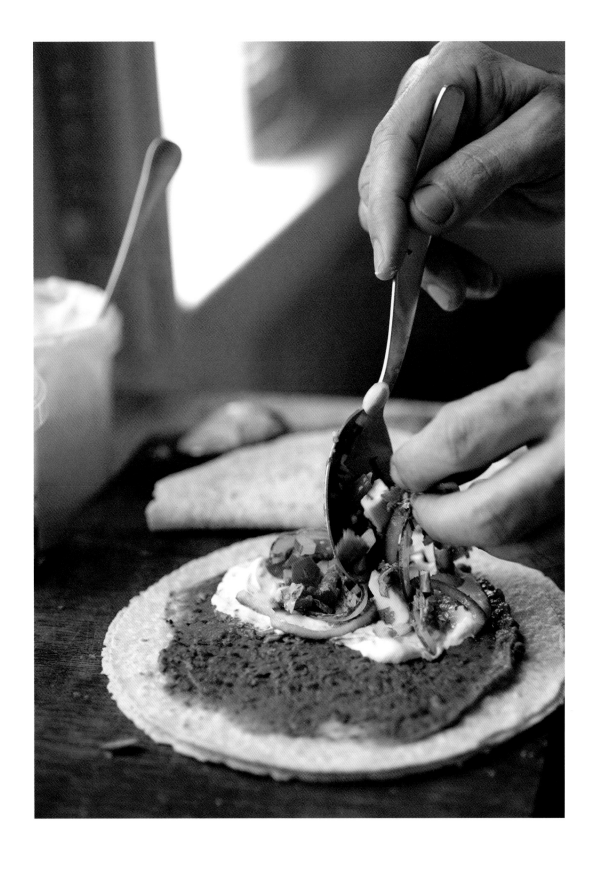

# Herb-stuffed tomatoes

This Provençal-style starter is quick to prepare. Serve it with a little salad of seasonal leaves and a few broken pieces of robust goat cheese.

Serves 4 as a small starter
4 medium tomatoes (ripe but firm)
salt
1 large onion, finely chopped
2 garlic cloves, finely chopped
12 wrinkly black olives, pitted and
    roughly chopped
2 tbsp olive oil
¼ cup panko
2 tbsp chopped oregano
3 tbsp chopped parsley
1 tbsp chopped mint
1½ tbsp chopped capers
black pepper

Preheat the oven to 325°F. Trim off about ⅜ inch from the top of each tomato and discard. Use a little spoon or a melon baller to remove the seeds and most of the flesh, leaving a clean shell. Lightly salt the inside of the tomatoes and place upside down in a colander, to drain off some moisture.

Meanwhile, put the onion, garlic, olives and 1 tablespoon of the oil in a medium pan and cook on low heat for 5 to 6 minutes, to soften the onion completely. Remove from the heat and stir in the panko, herbs, capers and some pepper. Taste and add salt, if you like.

Wipe the insides of the tomatoes with a paper towel, then fill them up with the herb stuffing, pressing down very gently as you go. You want a nice dome of stuffing on top.

Place the tomatoes in a greased ovenproof dish and drizzle lightly with the remaining oil. Bake for 35 to 45 minutes, or until the tomatoes soften. Serve hot or warm.

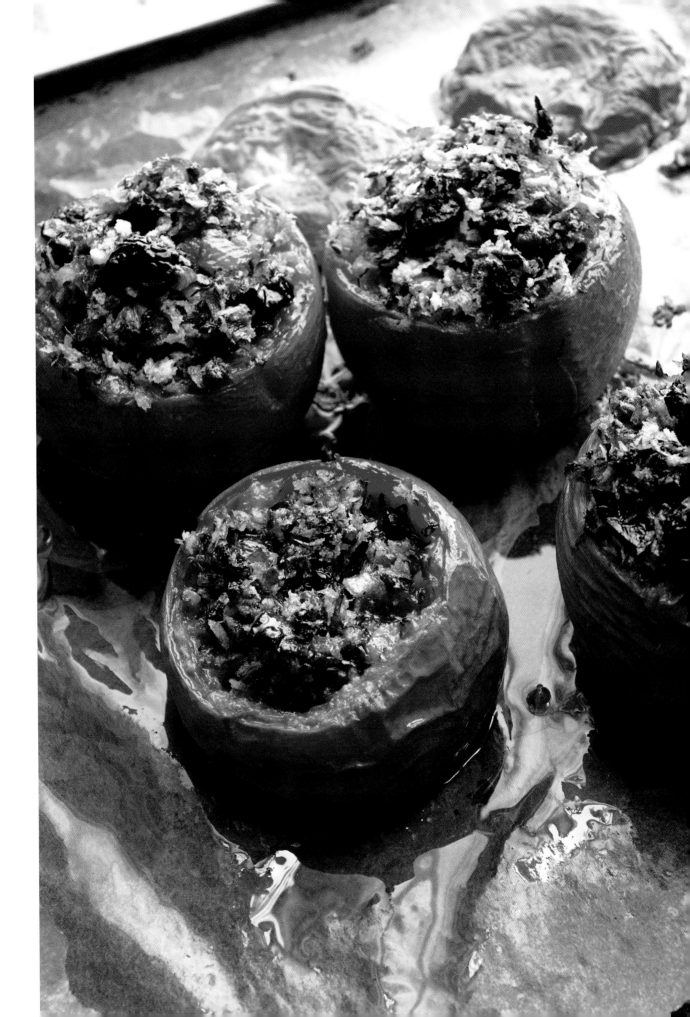

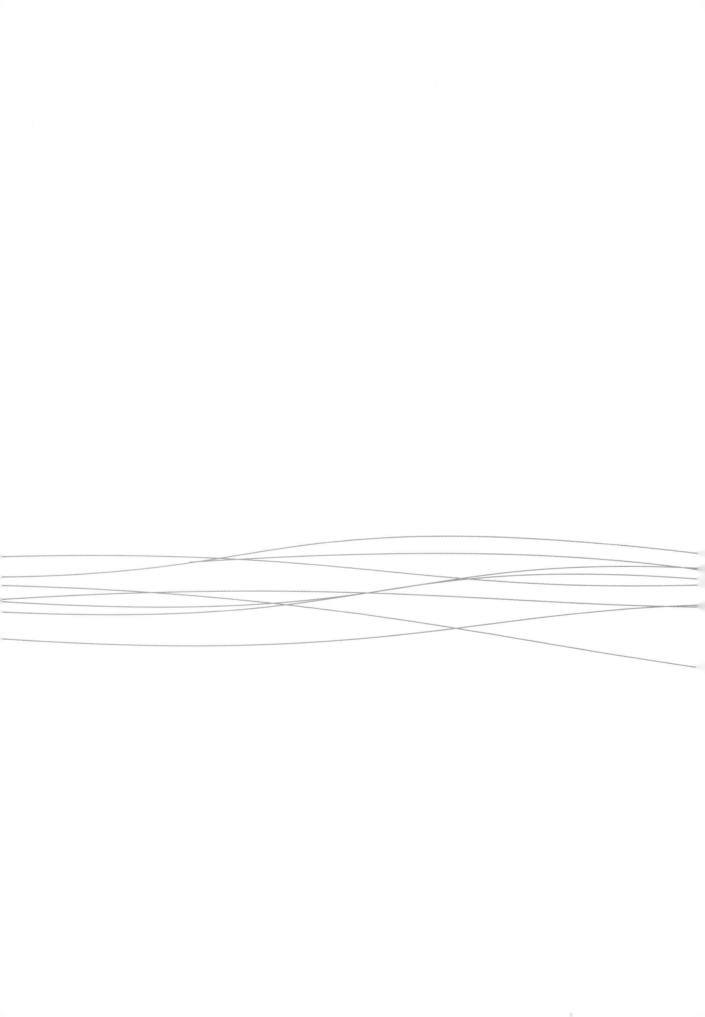

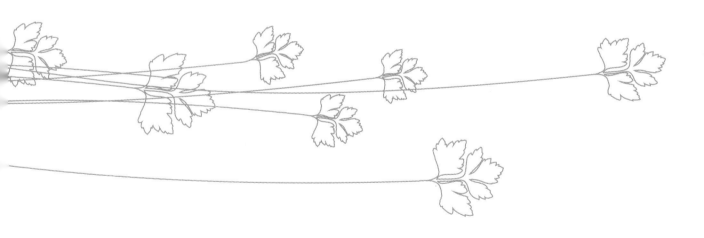

Leaves, Cooked and Raw

# Baked eggs with yogurt and chile

Here's my idea of comfort food and a perfect Sunday brunch treat. It is inspired by *çılbır*, which is Turkish poached eggs with yogurt. It calls for *kırmızı biber*, a common Turkish spice made from crushed chiles that have been rubbed with oil and often roasted. The Turks use it as a general condiment and also add it to melted butter to give the final touch to many dishes. *Kırmızı biber* has a sweet aroma and can vary in spiciness. You can get it from Turkish grocers or kalustyans.com. Alternatively, use plain chile flakes mixed with some sweet paprika.

Serves 2
¾ lb (about 14 cups) arugula
2 tbsp olive oil
salt
4 eggs
¾ cup Greek yogurt
1 garlic clove, crushed
4 tbsp unsalted butter
½ tsp *kırmızı biber*
6 sage leaves, shredded

Preheat the oven to 300°F. Place the arugula and oil in a large pan, add some salt and sauté on a medium heat for about 5 minutes, or until the arugula wilts and most of the liquid has evaporated.

Transfer to a small ovenproof dish and make four deep indentations in the arugula. Carefully break an egg into each hollow, taking care not to break the yolk. Place in the oven to cook for 10 to 15 minutes, or until the egg whites are set. (Alternatively, divide the arugula into small pans and cook two eggs in each.)

While the eggs are in the oven, mix the yogurt with the garlic and a pinch of salt. Stir well and set aside; do not chill.

Melt the butter in a small saucepan. Add the *kırmızı biber* and a pinch of salt and fry for 1 to 2 minutes, or until the butter starts to foam and turns a nice golden-red. Add the sage and cook for a few more seconds. Remove from the heat.

Once the eggs are cooked take them out of the oven. Spoon the yogurt over the center, and pour the hot chile butter over the yogurt and eggs. Serve immediately.

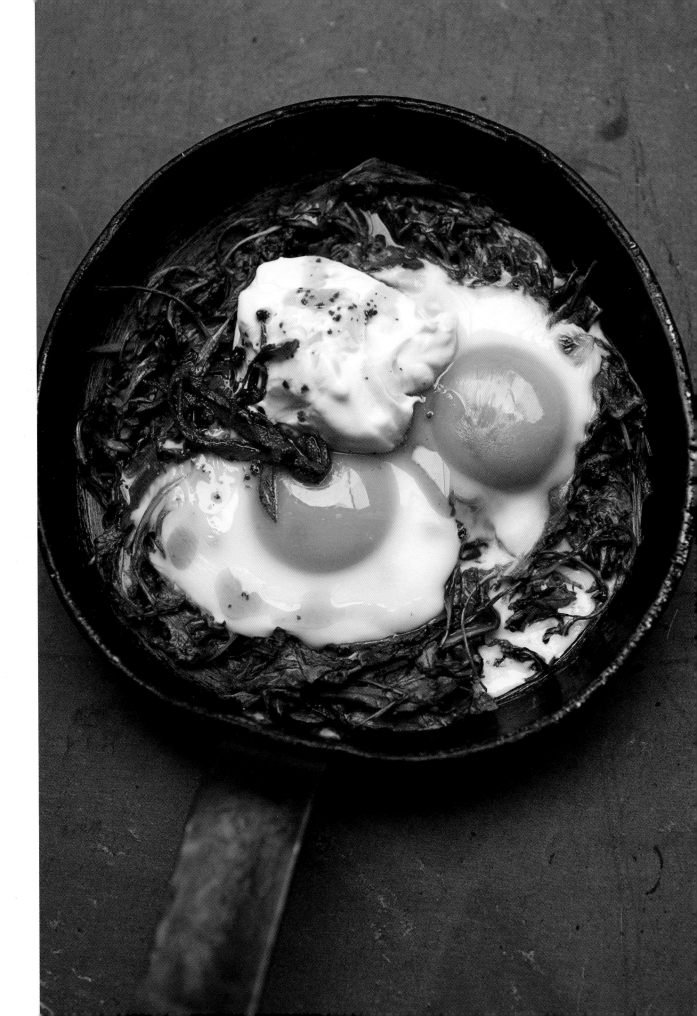

# Chard and saffron omelettes

Anybody who's been following my writing couldn't help noticing how much I carry on about chard. These wonderful leaves belong to the same family as beets. When picked small they make a great contribution to leafy salads, both in flavor and with their magnificent red hue. But it is the large, mature deep-green leaves – with stalks ranging from white, to yellow, to red and orange – that I love so much. They are in season from June to August, and have a sharp and earthy flavor, not too dominant but perfectly recognizable.

Both chard stalks and leaves are edible, although the stalks normally take a bit longer to cook. In most cases I slice the stalks thinly and the leaves a bit wider, then throw the stalks into a pan and sauté or blanch for 3 minutes before adding the leaves and cooking through. Here, though, I start them off together as they are cooked for a long time anyway.

Serves 4
½ lb (1 medium) waxy potato, peeled and cut into ⅜-inch dice
1 cup water
pinch of saffron threads
¾ lb Swiss chard (stalks and leaves), shredded
salt and pepper
2 tbsp lemon juice
1 garlic clove, crushed
5 eggs
¼ cup milk
⅔ cup chopped herbs (tarragon, dill, parsley)
vegetable oil
½ cup crème fraîche, cold

Put the potatoes, water and saffron in a large pan and bring to the boil. Simmer for 4 minutes, then add the chard and some salt and pepper. Continue cooking, covered, for 10 to 15 minutes, or until the potato is soft. Drain out any excess liquid that is left in the pan. Off the heat, add the lemon juice and garlic. Leave to cool.

Whisk together well the eggs, milk, herbs and some salt and pepper. Pour 1 teaspoon of oil into a hot, 9-inch nonstick frying pan, then use one-quarter of the egg mix to make a thin round omelette. Transfer to paper towels. Make three more omelettes in the same way. Leave to cool down.

Divide the cold crème fraîche among the omelettes, spreading it over one half of each. Taste the chard mix and adjust the seasoning, then spread generously over the crème fraîche. Fold each omelette over in half, then fold again to get a fan shape. Allow the chard mix to show at the open side. Arrange the omelettes in a lightly oiled ovenproof dish or on a baking sheet. (Keep in the fridge if making ahead.) When ready to serve, preheat the oven to 325°F. Place the omelettes in the oven for 5 to 8 minutes, or until hot. Serve at once.

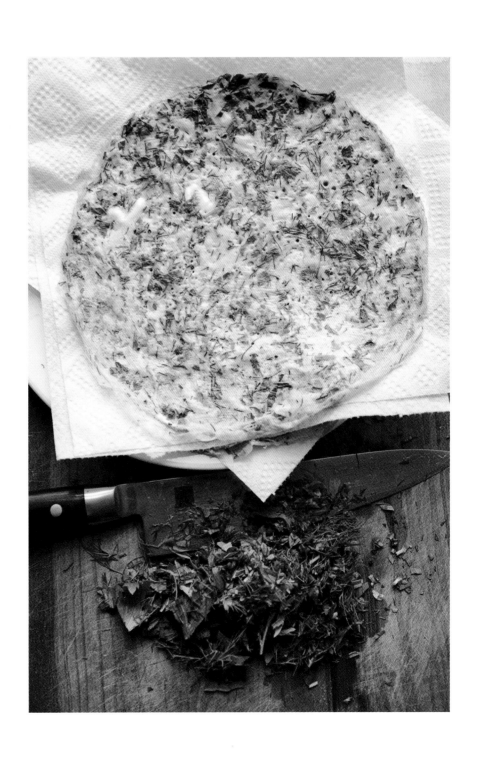

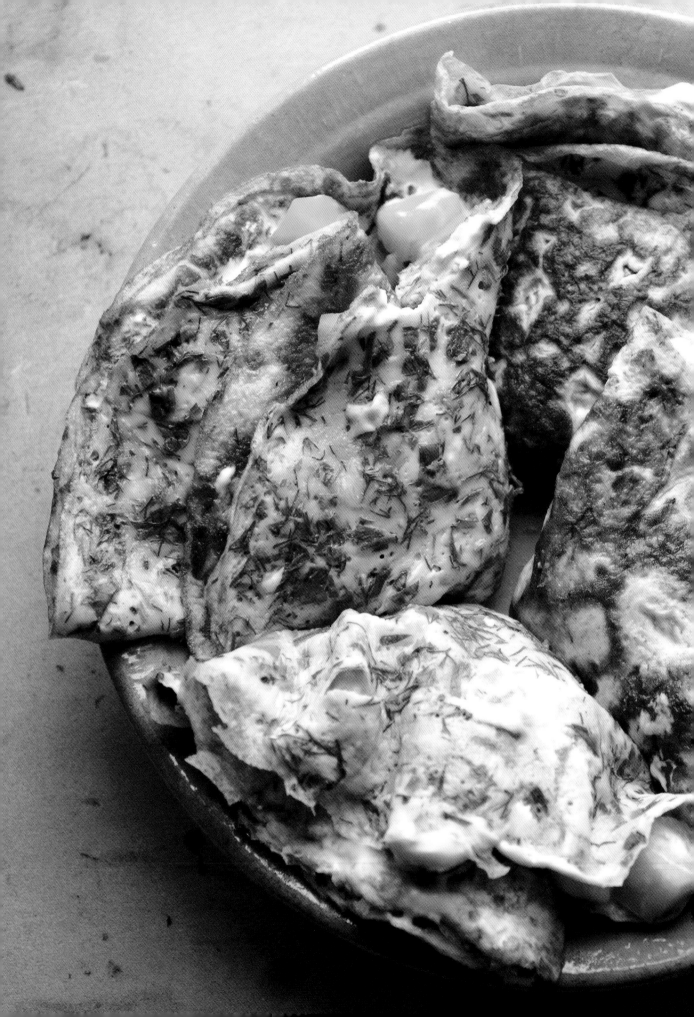

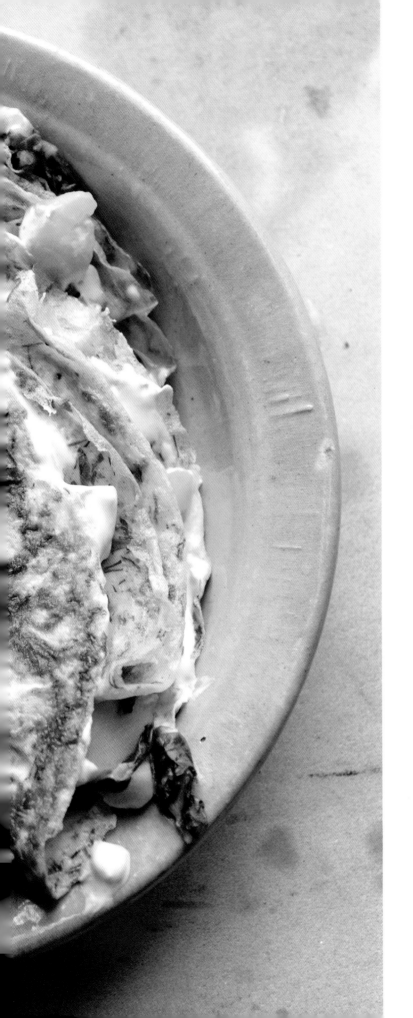

# Lettuce salad

It is essential for every good cook to have a solid lettuce salad up their sleeve, a good in-between course to cleanse the palate and lighten the spirits. This one should do the trick; it also makes for a good starter.

I am not very fond of sun-dried tomatoes, particularly not for salads – they are harsh, both in flavor and texture – but I love semi-dried tomatoes. You can make them yourself (see Castelluccio Lentils with Tomatoes and Gorgonzola, page 222) and store in olive oil for quite some time, or buy one of the commercial varieties that go by funny names such as "sun-blushed" or "sun-kissed."

Serves 4
**Dressing**
1 garlic clove, crushed
1½ tbsp lemon juice
1½ tbsp olive oil
1 tbsp grapeseed oil
salt and black pepper

1 head of butter lettuce, leaves
    separated
½ head of curly lettuce, leaves
    separated
1 head of radicchio, leaves separated
3 green onions, green and white parts,
    sliced thinly on a sharp angle
20 radishes, trimmed and cut into
    ⅛-inch-thick slices
2 cups semi-dried tomatoes, whole or
    roughly torn
2 tbsp capers, whole if small or very
    roughly chopped

To make the dressing. In a small bowl whisk together the ingredients, being quite generous with the salt and pepper.

Wash the lettuce leaves, dry well and keep whole or tear into large pieces. Place in a large mixing bowl and add the radicchio, green onions, radishes and tomatoes.

Just before serving, pour the dressing over the salad and toss gently. Transfer to a large mixing bowl and sprinkle the capers over the top.

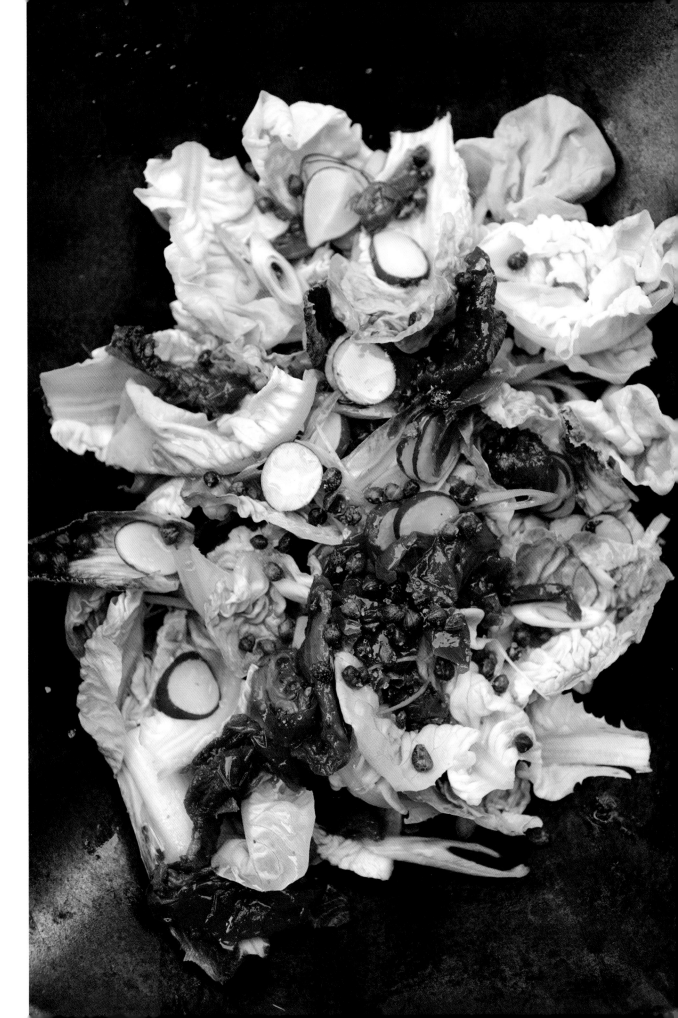

# Swiss chard, chickpea and tamarind stew

I always want to add sharpness to slow-cooked, stewy-type dishes, something to break down the heavy seriousness of the dish and introduce a little refreshing edge to it – a bit of humor even. The Italians invented gremolata – chopped garlic, parsley and lemon zest – which they use to finish off the famous *ossobuco alla milanese*. Here, though, I don't really need this kind of thing as I include heaps of sharpness in the dish from the start, in the form of tamarind and chard (for more on chard, see Chard and Saffron Omelettes on page 142). Still, I can't resist the temptation of a little lemon juice at the end, just in case; some chile flakes will also give it a kick if you want to add them. This is a perfect main course for when it gets a bit cloudy.

Serves 4

4 tbsp seedless tamarind pulp

1 lb Swiss chard (stalks and leaves), cut into ⅜-inch slices

1½ tsp coriander seeds

1 medium onion, thinly sliced

2 tsp caraway seeds

1½ tbsp olive oil, plus extra to finish

1 tsp tomato paste

one 14-oz can chopped plum tomatoes, with their juices

1½ cups water

1½ tbsp sugar

2½ cups freshly cooked chickpeas (or a 14-oz can, drained)

salt and black pepper

juice of 1 lemon

1 cup Greek yogurt (optional)

generous handful of cilantro leaves

1¾ cups short-grain rice

1½ tbsp butter

3 cups water

Start by whisking the tamarind with about 3 tablespoons of warm water until it dissolves into a paste. Set aside.

Bring a medium pot of salted water to the boil and blanch the chard for 2 minutes. Drain in a colander.

Dry-roast the coriander seeds in a small pan over medium heat, then grind to a powder with a mortar and pestle.

Next, put the onion, caraway seeds and olive oil in a large heavy pan and sauté on medium heat for about 10 minutes, or until the onion is soft and golden. Add the tomato paste and stir as you cook it for about a minute. Add the canned tomatoes, water, sugar, chickpeas, ground coriander, chard and some salt and pepper.

Strain the tamarind water through a small sieve into the pan. Bring to the boil, then cover with a lid and leave to simmer for about 30 minutes. When ready, the dish should have the consistency of a thick soup. You can adjust this either by adding more water or simmering uncovered so the excess liquid can evaporate. Taste and add more salt and pepper if needed.

While the stew is cooking, put the rice, butter and a bit of salt in a medium pan and set on a medium heat. Stir to coat the rice with butter. Add the water and bring to the boil, then cover the pan with a tight-fitting lid and leave to simmer on a low flame for 15 to 20 minutes. Remove from the heat and leave covered for 5 minutes.

When ready to serve, spoon the rice into shallow soup bowls, creating a large crater in the center. Add the lemon juice to the stew and stir, then put a ladle or two into the middle of the rice in each bowl. Spoon yogurt on top, if you like. Drizzle with oil and finish with plenty of cilantro leaves.

# Chard cakes with sorrel sauce

The cheese I use in these splendid cakes is *kashkaval*, of which there are different regional varieties all over the Balkans. There is also an Italian version called caciocavallo. Kashkaval is normally made from sheep's milk and has a tangy yet nutty flavor. You can get it from Arab or Turkish grocers (see Dates and Turkish Sheep's Cheese on page 280). Choose a strong and less industrialized variety. If you can't get it, replace with mature pecorino.

You don't necessarily have to make the sauce as the cakes work perfectly well accompanied with just a wedge of lemon. Still, if you choose to make it (and I can't recommend it enough) you'll be able to keep it in the fridge for a day or two and serve it with a million other things – roasted root vegetables, hearty lentils, red meat and oily fish. (For more on chard, see Chard and Saffron Omelettes, page 142.)

Serves 4 as a starter

Sauce

3 cups sorrel leaves, washed

½ cup Greek yogurt

1 garlic clove, crushed

2 tbsp olive oil

½ tsp Dijon mustard

salt

1¼ lbs Swiss chard

⅓ cup pine nuts

1 tbsp olive oil

4 oz kashkaval cheese, coarsely grated

1 egg

6 tbsp dried white breadcrumbs

¼ tsp salt

black pepper

half-and-half vegetable oil and olive oil
    for frying

To make the sauce. Place all the ingredients in a food processor or a blender and blitz to a fine bright-green sauce. Taste and adjust the amount of salt. Keep in the fridge until needed.

Cut the woody white stalks from the green chard leaves. Bring a large pan of water to the boil. Add the stalks and simmer for 4 minutes. Then add the leaves, stir and continue simmering for 3 minutes. Drain the chard and allow to cool down slightly. Once cool enough to handle, squeeze as much water out of the chard as possible. You need to use both hands and be quite forceful to do this. Next, chop the leaves and stalks roughly and put in a mixing bowl.

In a small pan fry the pine nuts in the tablespoon of olive oil for 1 minute, or until light brown (watch out; they darken in seconds). Add the nuts and oil to the chard, followed by the cheese, egg, breadcrumbs, salt and some pepper. If the mix is very soft and sticky you might need to add more crumbs.

Pour enough frying oil into a frying pan to come ¼ inch up the sides. Shape the chard mix into eight patties that are roughly 2 inches in diameter and ⅝ inch thick. Fry them for about 3 minutes on each side, or until golden brown. Transfer onto paper towels to absorb the oil. Serve warm or at room temperature, with the sauce on the side.

# Green pancakes with lime butter

This recipe brought lots of compliments round my way after I first published it in 2008. I guess these pancakes are so comforting they somehow take you back to your childhood, when the joy of textures and flavors is still pure and unadulterated. Brunch is the ideal meal for them, served with a salad of seasonal leaves and possibly also a slice of freshly grilled halloumi or a piece of smoked fish.

Some lime butter will probably be left over. Keep it in the fridge and then smear it over a baked sweet potato.

Serves 3–4

**Lime butter**

8 tbsp (1 stick) unsalted butter, at room temperature
grated zest of 1 lime
1½ tbsp lime juice
¼ tsp salt
½ tsp white pepper
1 tbsp chopped cilantro
½ garlic clove, finely chopped
¼ tsp chile flakes

½ lb (about 8 cups) spinach, washed
¾ cup self-rising flour (see page 28)
1 tbsp baking powder
1 egg
4 tbsp unsalted butter, melted
½ tsp salt
1 tsp ground cumin
⅔ cup milk
6 medium green onions, finely sliced
2 fresh green chiles, thinly sliced
1 egg white
olive oil for frying

To make the lime butter. Put the butter in a medium bowl and beat it with a wooden spoon until it turns soft and creamy. Stir in the rest of the ingredients. Tip onto a sheet of plastic wrap and roll into a sausage shape. Twist the ends of the wrap to seal the flavored butter. Chill until firm.

Wilt the spinach in a pan with a splash of water. Drain in a sieve and, when cool, squeeze hard with your hands to remove as much moisture as possible. Roughly chop and put aside.

Put the flour, baking powder, whole egg, melted butter, salt, cumin and milk in a large mixing bowl and whisk until smooth. Add the green onions, chiles and spinach and mix with a fork. Whisk the egg white to soft peaks and gently fold it into the batter.

Pour a small amount of olive oil into a heavy frying pan and place on medium–high heat. For each pancake, ladle 2 tablespoons of batter into the pan and press down gently. You should get smallish pancakes, about 3 inches in diameter and ⅜ inch thick. Cook for about 2 minutes on each side, or until you get a good golden-green color. Transfer to paper towels and keep warm. Continue making pancakes, adding oil to the pan as needed, until the batter is used up.

To serve, pile up three warm pancakes per person and place a slice of flavored butter on top to melt.

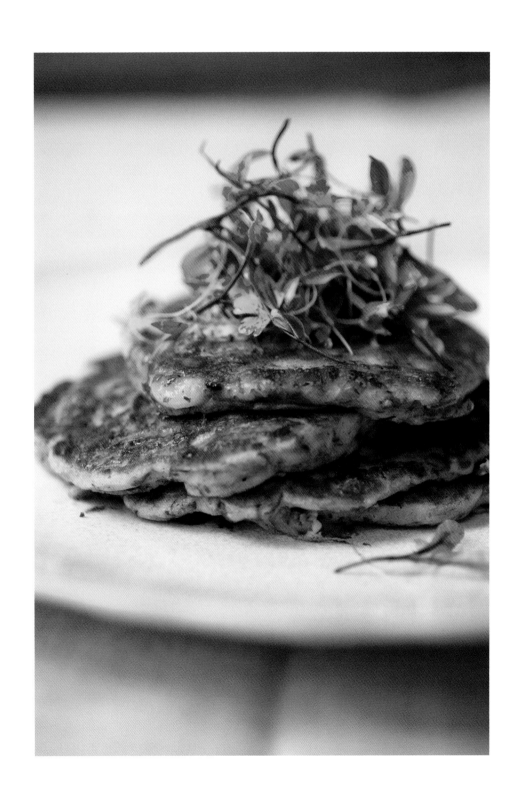

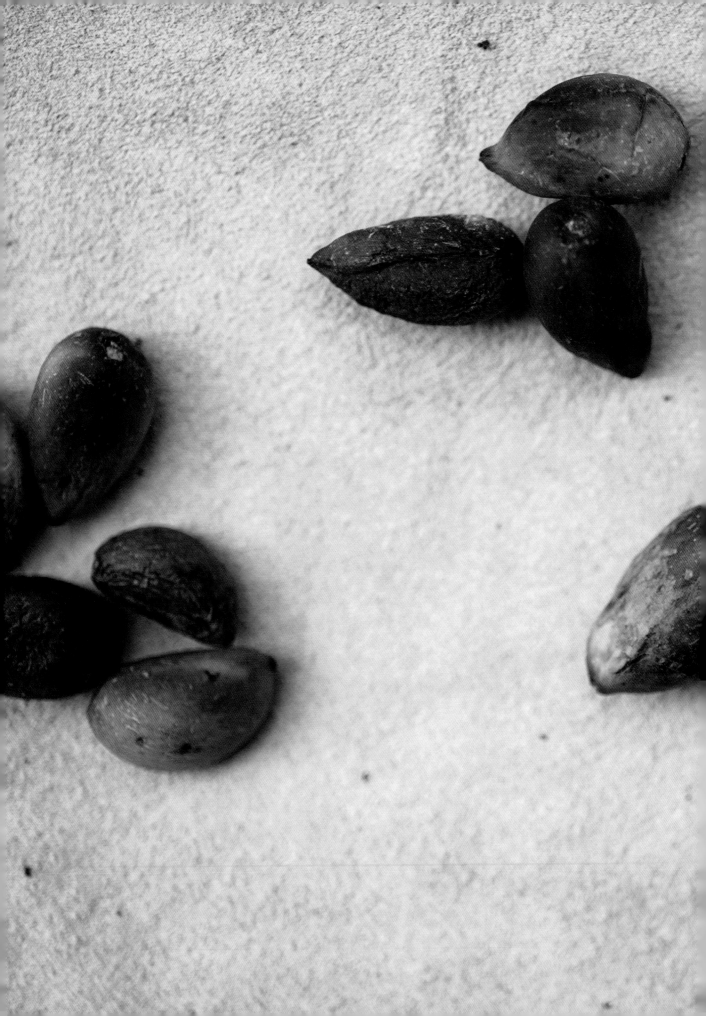

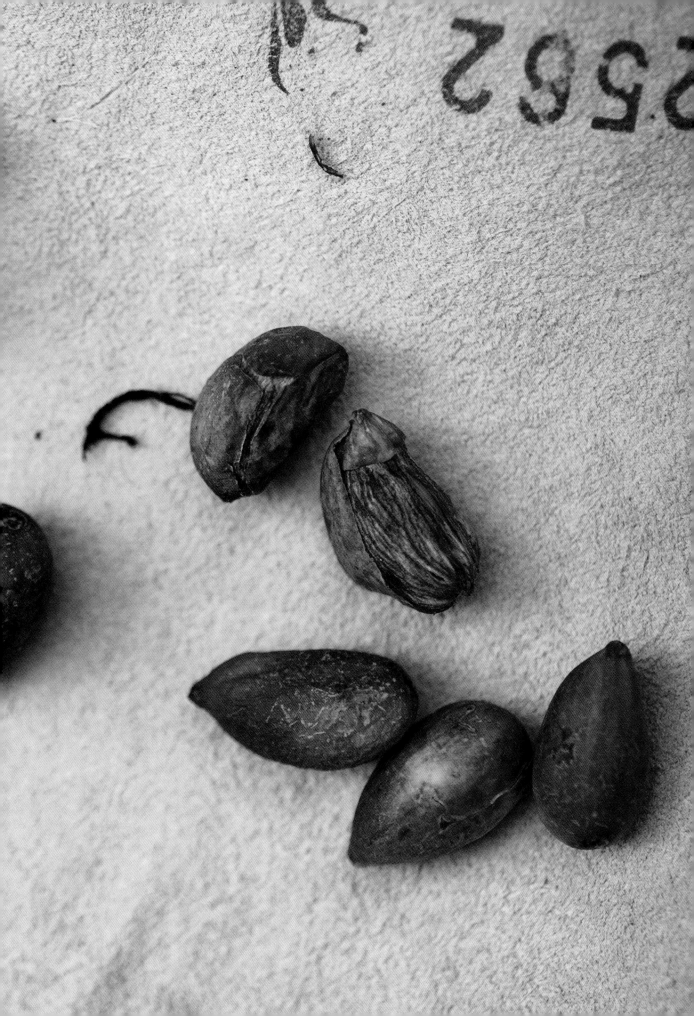

# Watercress, pistachio and orange blossom salad

I would either start a meal or end it with this salad. It is an ideal palate-cleanser with its robust yet refreshing herb flavors. Or, you could serve it to balance a long-cooked or rich main course, such as the Smoky frittata on page 96. Another idea is to add spoonfuls of buffalo ricotta to transform the salad into a more substantial starter.

It is essential to dress the salad as you serve it and not a second earlier: the delicate herbs wilt in an instant when they come in contact with the acidic dressing.

Serves 4

**Dressing**

4 tbsp olive oil

1½ tbsp lemon juice (or more if you like it very sour)

1 tsp orange-flower water

salt and black pepper

3½ cups watercress, thick stalks removed

scant 1 cup basil leaves

1½ cups cilantro leaves

¼ cup dill

¼ cup tarragon leaves

⅓ cup shelled unsalted pistachios, lightly toasted and coarsely crushed

To make the dressing. In a little bowl whisk together all of the dressing ingredients.

Place the watercress and herbs in a large mixing bowl and set aside until you are ready to serve the salad (you can leave them in the fridge in an airtight container for a few hours).

Just before serving, pour the dressing and the pistachios over the leaves, toss gently and serve immediately.

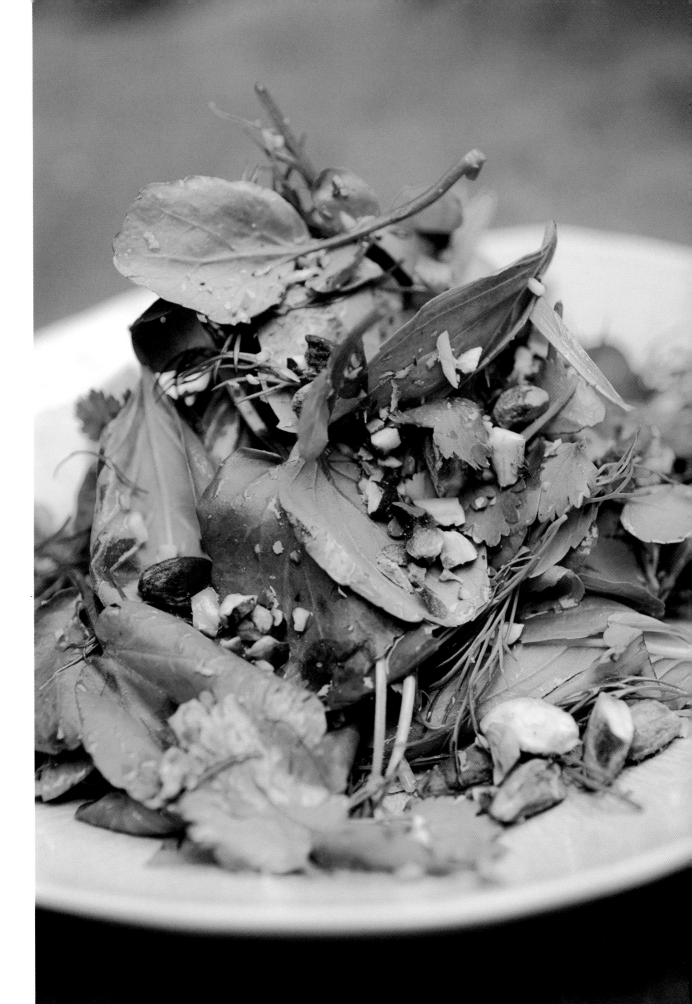

# Egg, spinach and pecorino pizza

This started off as a take on *manakish*, a Levantine flatbread topped with za'atar and often also containing halloumi-style cheese or minced lamb. My version is so far removed from the original that it doesn't warrant the use of the name. Still, the za'atar and sumac give this "pizza" an earthy Middle Eastern kick, reminiscent of the aromas coming from bread stalls in East Jerusalem. (For information on za'atar and sumac, see Fried Lima Beans with Feta, Sorrel and Sumac, page 214.)

You'll probably find it difficult to fit the six individual pizzas into your oven all at once: you'd need three baking sheets large enough to take two pizzas each. If you haven't got them, bake the individual pizzas in batches or make three double-sized pizzas.

Serves 6 (makes 6 individual pizzas)

2½ tsp dried yeast

1¾ cups tepid water (no hotter than 86°F)

5½ cups white bread flour, plus extra for dusting

1¼ tsp salt

⅔ cup olive oil

2 lbs spinach, washed

1 lb pecorino, grated

1½ tbsp sumac

1½ tbsp za'atar

coarse salt and black pepper

6 eggs

Dissolve the yeast in the water. Add to the flour together with the salt and 2 tablespoons of the olive oil. Knead by hand or in a heavy electric mixer for 8 to 10 minutes, adding a little bit more flour if the dough is sticky; it should become smooth and silky. Brush a large bowl with a bit of oil, put the dough inside and cover with a wet towel. Leave to rise in a warmish place for 1 to 2 hours, or until the dough doubles in size.

When ready, divide the dough into six similarly sized pieces. Use a rolling pin to roll each into a disc that is roughly ¼ inch thick and 7 inches in diameter. Transfer to baking sheets dusted with a bit of flour and leave to rise again in a warm place for about 30 minutes.

Preheat the oven to 400°F. Wilt the spinach in a large saucepan with 4 tablespoons of the olive oil. Allow to cool down, then squeeze out all the liquid from the spinach.

Scatter the cheese evenly over the pizza bases and spread the spinach over this, making a slight well in the center to break the egg into later on. Sprinkle the sumac, za'atar and black pepper on top. Drizzle about 1½ teaspoons olive oil over each pizza.

Bake for 12 to 15 minutes, or until the crust turns a nice brown. Remove from the oven and quickly break a whole egg into the center of each pizza. Use a fork to spread the white around, keeping the yolk whole. Sprinkle with coarse salt and return to the oven to bake for 5 minutes, or just until the whites set but the yolks are still runny. Serve at once.

# Caramelized endive with Gruyère

When I first published this recipe in the *Guardian* in 2007 I used Taleggio and was perfectly happy with it. Still, when I tried the dish again for this book I decided to double-check which cheese variety worked best. Taleggio (See Stuffed Portobello with Melting Taleggio, page 56) was a winner for its creaminess and its ability to penetrate in between the endive leaves. But I chose Gruyère in the end because its piquant flavor works better with the endive's bitterness. You can now make your choice. Another, less cheesy option is raclette, which was born to melt.

Serves 4
1 tbsp olive oil
1½ tbsp butter
½ tsp sugar
salt
4 endives, cut in half lengthways
2 tsp thyme leaves, finely chopped
7 oz Gruyère, sliced
1½ tsp fresh breadcrumbs
black pepper

Preheat the oven to 375°F. Place a heavy, flat pan on medium heat. Add the oil, butter, sugar and a pinch of salt, and allow to heat up.

Place the endive halves, cut-side down, in the pan. Do not move them for 3 to 5 minutes, or until they turn deep golden. (You might need to do this in two batches as the endives need space.) Remove from the heat. Transfer the endive halves to a small ovenproof dish, arranging them cut-side up, close together. Sprinkle with half the thyme. Place the slices of cheese on top and sprinkle with the rest of the thyme.

Place in the oven to bake for 8 to 12 minutes, or until the cheese starts to bubble. Remove from the oven. Sprinkle with the breadcrumbs and some black pepper. Return to the oven, increase the temperature to 400°F and bake for 5 to 7 minutes, or until the breadcrumbs brown. Serve hot.

# Grape leaf, herb and yogurt pie

Whenever I walk into a bookshop I find myself in the cookery section within seconds; it's an urge I can't control. On a recent visit to a secondhand bookshop in Hay-on-Wye, the capital of bookshops, I came across a real treasure, *Classic Turkish Cookery* by Ghillie Başan, published in 1995. This book offers a fantastic introduction to one of the world's most accomplished cuisines and it is packed full of recipes you just know you must try. It is there that I came across this unusual savory cake originating from the Turkish part of Cyprus. It makes a substantial snack or a light starter. Serve with Burnt Eggplant with Tahini (page 122).

Serves 4

20 to 25 grape leaves (fresh or from a jar)
4 shallots, finely chopped
4 tbsp olive oil
1½ tbsp unsalted butter, melted
1 cup Greek yogurt, plus extra to serve
2½ tbsp pine nuts, lightly toasted
½ tbsp finely chopped tarragon
2 tbsp finely chopped parsley
3 tbsp finely chopped dill
4 tbsp finely chopped mint
grated zest of 1 lemon
1 tbsp lemon juice
salt and black pepper
½ cup rice flour
3 tbsp dried breadcrumbs (preferably panko)

Preheat the oven to 375°F. Place the grape leaves in a shallow bowl, cover with boiling water and leave for 10 minutes. Then remove the leaves from the water and dry them well with a tea towel. Use scissors to trim off and discard the bit of hard stalk at the base of each leaf.

Sauté the shallots in 1 tablespoon of the oil for about 8 minutes, or until light brown. Leave to cool down.

Take a round and shallow ovenproof dish that is roughly 8 inches in diameter, and cover its bottom and sides with grape leaves, slightly overlapping them and allowing the leaves to hang over the rim of the dish. Mix the melted butter with 2 tablespoons of olive oil; use about two-thirds of this to generously brush the leaves lining the dish.

Mix together in a bowl the shallots, yogurt, pine nuts, chopped herbs and lemon zest and juice, and season with salt and pepper to taste. Then add the rice flour and mix well until you get a homogenous paste. Spread this paste evenly in the baking dish.

Fold the overhanging grape leaves back over the top of the filling so they cover the edges, then cover the filling completely with the remaining grape leaves. Brush with the rest of the butter and oil mix. Finally, scatter the breadcrumbs over the top and drizzle over the remaining 1 tablespoon olive oil.

Bake for 40 minutes, or until the leaves crisp up and the breadcrumbs turn golden brown. Remove from the oven and leave to rest for at least 10 minutes. Cut into wedges and serve warmish or at room temperature, with a dollop of fresh yogurt.

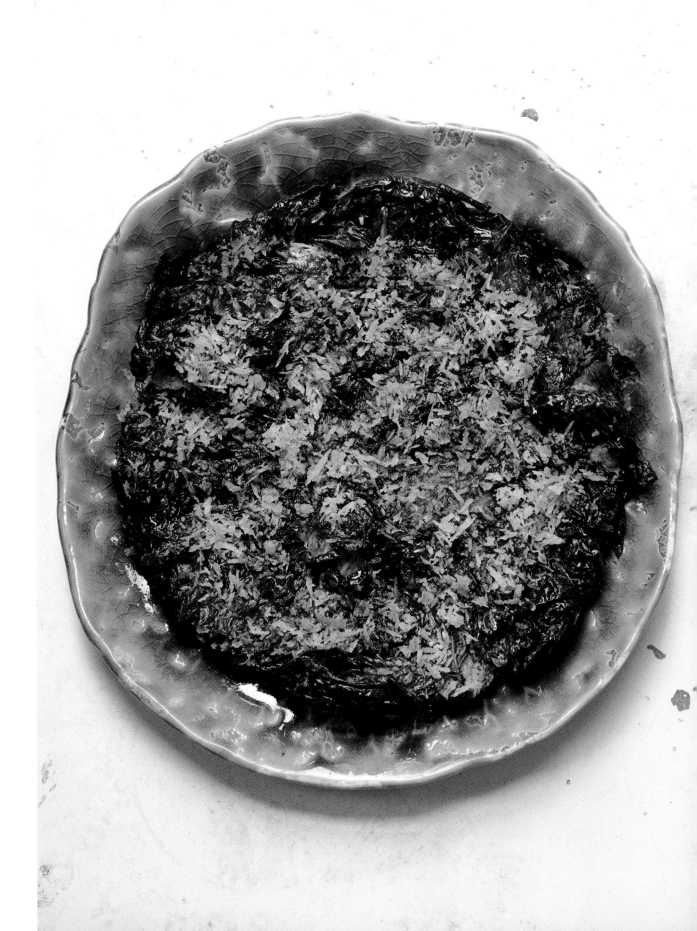

# Nutty endive with Roquefort

You really need to get your hands dirty here. The flavored crème fraîche has to cover every bit of endive leaf in order to flavor it properly, because endive's fresh, watery and slightly bitter nature asks for a lot of rich dressing. On top of that I add butter-toasted nuts, a welcome addition to almost any salad, to make this a truly sumptuous starter.

A note about Roquefort and other European cheeses: as a general rule, most continental cheeses use rennet, a cluster of enzymes taken from animals' stomachs that causes milk to coagulate and eventually form into cheese. British cheeses tend to be based on vegetarian alternatives to rennet. Here, as in all recipes with cheese, I encourage a strict vegetarian to check thoroughly whether the variety is completely vegetarian and, if not, to look for alternatives; these can often be found online.

Serves 4 as a starter

1¾ oz Roquefort or another strong
   blue cheese
¾ cup crème fraîche
white pepper
⅓ cup roughly chopped pine nuts
⅓ cup roughly chopped walnuts
1 tsp butter
salt
2 endives
a few leaves of radicchio, Treviso or
   baby chard

Grate the Roquefort on a coarse grater and place in a bowl with the crème fraîche and some white pepper. Use a whisk to mix thoroughly to a thick mixture. Taste and adjust the seasoning.

In a hot frying pan lightly toast the nuts with the butter and pinch of salt. Keep shaking the pan to get an even golden color on all the nuts. Leave to cool.

Trim the base of the endives and pick off the outer leaves. Trim a bit more to remove more leaves until you get to the core. Using your hands, smear each leaf with plenty of the Roquefort mix. Form bundles of six to eight leaves pressed together, each leaf partly encased in a larger one.

Line a serving dish with some red leaves. Place a few bundles of endive on top, stacking them or leaning them standing against each other. Sprinkle generously with the toasted nuts and serve.

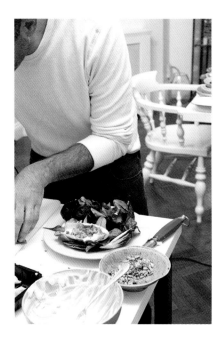

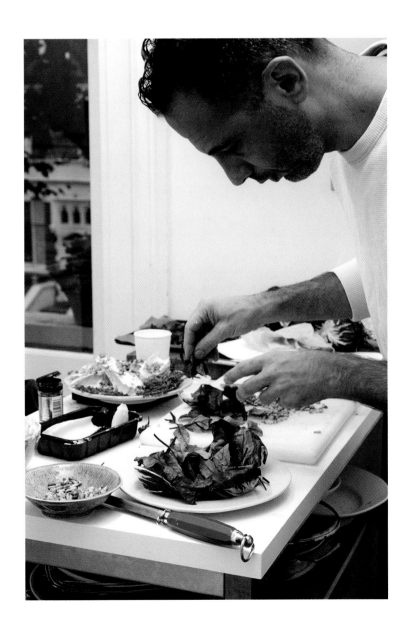
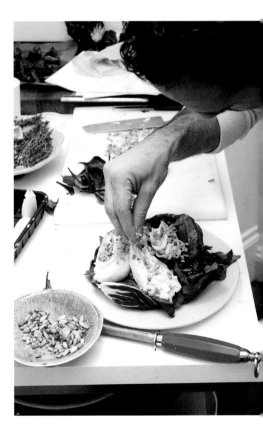

# Bittersweet salad

I don't usually celebrate Valentine's Day. This is due to cowardly cynicism, combined with a firm belief that you cannot just create a momentous intimate occasion, especially when millions of other couples are trying to do exactly the same. It just feels a bit claustrophobic. But if you twisted my arm and forced me to, I guess I would choose this salad to celebrate the day, representing the more realistic flavors of love: bitter and sweet.

The theme here is red. For this salad I'd go out of my way to find an exciting combination of red leaves and herbs. I love the long, twisted red leaves of some varieties of radicchio di Treviso. Red orach, purple basil, red amaranth and bull's blood (red) chard are also stunning leaves. Some tiny sprouting varieties, such as radish or purple basil, will also add character.

Serves 2 (of course)
2 blood oranges (or plain oranges)
blood orange juice as needed
1¼ tbsp lemon juice
¼ cup maple syrup
coarse sea salt
½ tsp orange-flower water
½ small radicchio
1 small Treviso, leaves separated
1 tbsp olive oil
black pepper
handful of small red leaves
¾ cup good-quality ricotta
2 tbsp pine nuts, toasted
seeds from 1 small pomegranate
    (see page 110)

Take each of the blood oranges in turn and use a small sharp knife to slice off the top and base. Now cut down the side of the orange, following its natural curve, to remove the skin and white pith. Over a small bowl, cut in between the membranes to remove the individual segments into the bowl. Squeeze all the juice from the membrane and skin into a small saucepan.

Make up the juice in the pan to 7 tbsp with extra blood orange juice. Add the lemon juice, maple syrup and a pinch of salt and bring to a light simmer. Leave to reduce for 20 to 25 minutes, or until you are left with about 3 tablespoons of thick syrup. Strain it through a fine sieve and allow to cool down, then stir in the orange-flower water.

Pull apart the radicchio leaves and tear them roughly into large pieces. Put into a mixing bowl. Add the Treviso leaves, oil and some salt and pepper, and toss gently. Divide the salad leaves between two serving plates. Dot with the orange segments, small red leaves and spoonfuls of ricotta, building the salad up. Drizzle with the orange syrup and finish with pine nuts and pomegranate seeds.

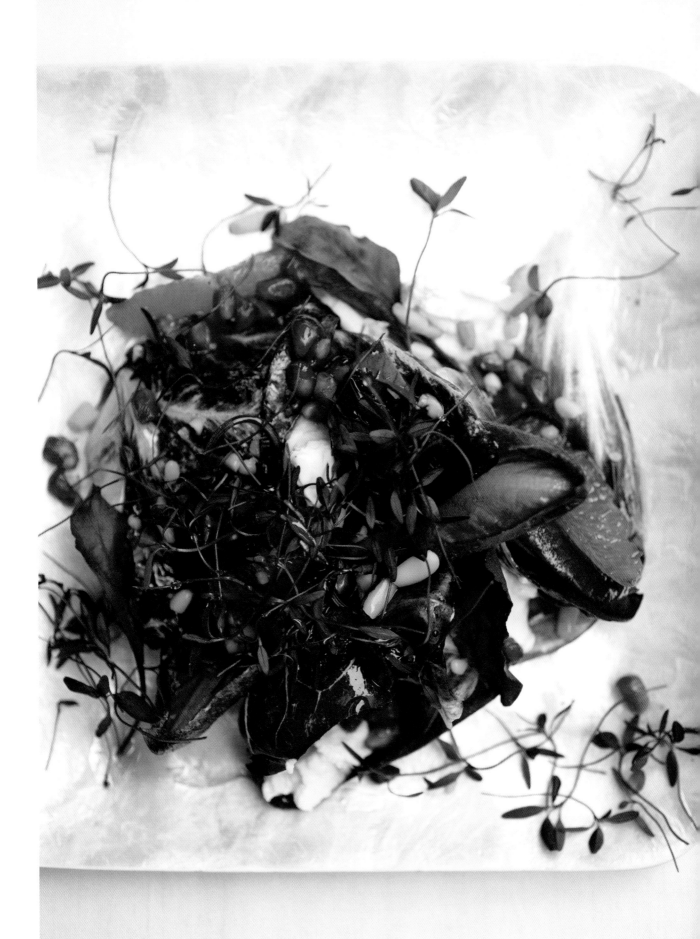

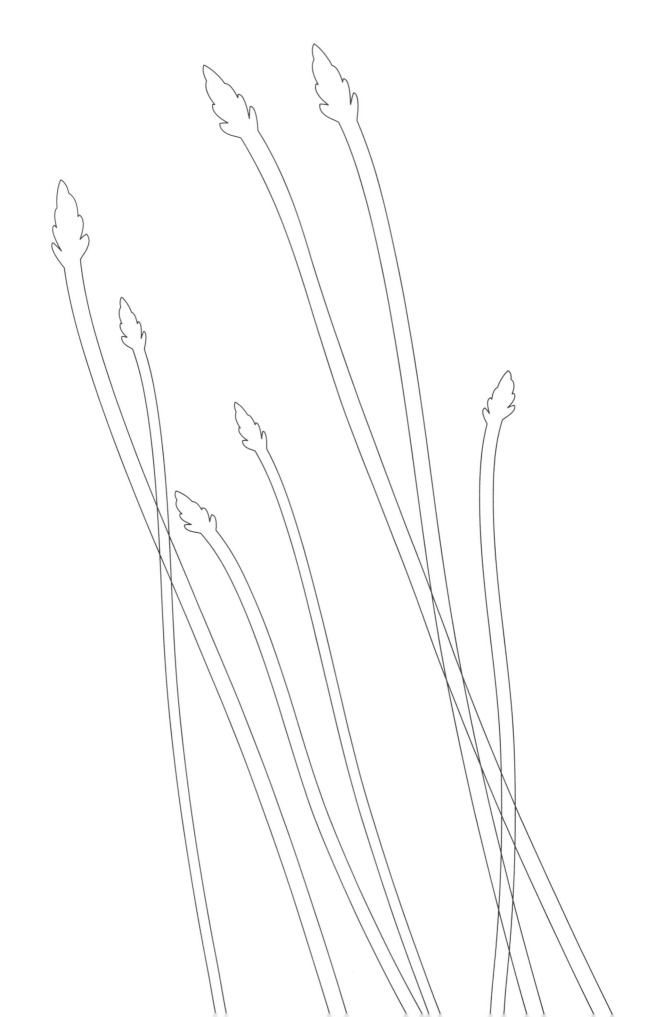

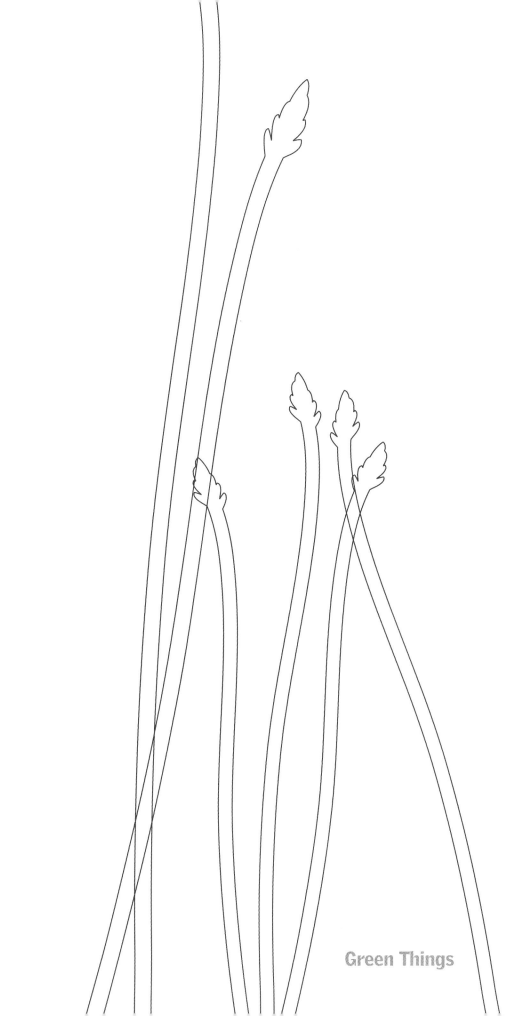

Green Things

# Cucumber salad with smashed garlic and ginger

I have a terrible habit of adding yogurt or sour cream to almost anything that's been cooking for a long time, has got a lot of heat, is slightly greasy or just seems a bit heavy to me. Terrible – because I know not everyone is keen on adding dairy products left, right and center, particularly not to a perfectly nice dish of pulses, a spicy vegetable stew or a roasted cut of lean meat. So here's a perfect alternative, a dish shouting freshness that would go well with plenty of hearty dishes. Try it with Sweet Potato Cakes (page 32) or with Coconut Rice with Sambal and Okra (page 230).

Serves 4–6 as a condiment or a side
dish

**Dressing**

3 tbsp rice wine vinegar

2 tsp sugar

2 tbsp sunflower oil

2 tsp toasted sesame oil

1 small red onion, very thinly sliced

1½ inches fresh ginger, peeled and
sliced

1 tsp Maldon sea salt

2 large garlic cloves, peeled

4 small (or 8 mini) cucumbers (1¼ lbs),
peeled

1 tbsp toasted sesame seeds

3 tbsp chopped cilantro

To make the dressing. Whisk together all the dressing ingredients in a medium mixing bowl.

Add the sliced red onion, mix well and leave aside to marinate for about an hour.

Place the ginger and salt in a mortar and pound well with a pestle. Add the garlic and continue pounding until it is also well crushed and broken into pieces (stop pounding before it disintegrates into a paste). Use a spatula to scrape the contents of the mortar into the bowl with the onion and dressing. Stir together.

Cut the cucumbers lengthways in half, then cut each half on an angle into ¼-inch-thick slices. Add the cucumber to the bowl, followed by the sesame seeds and cilantro. Stir well and leave to sit for 10 minutes.

Before serving, stir the salad again, tip out some of the liquid that has accumulated at the bottom of the bowl and adjust the seasoning.

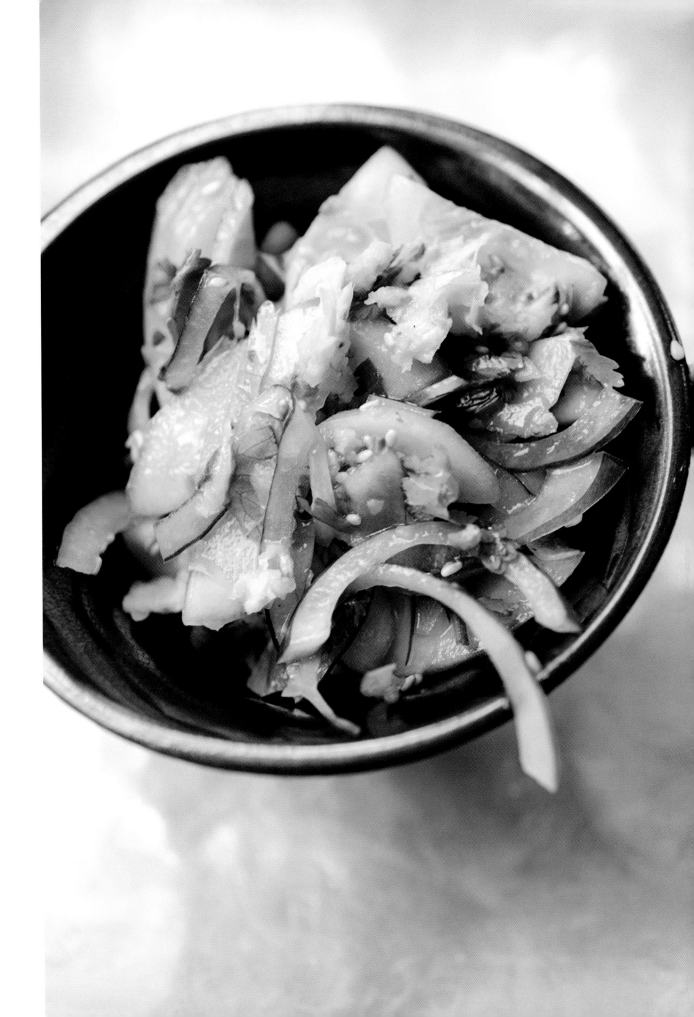

# Lemony globe artichokes

This is a majestic dish, perfect for starting off a light summer's supper. Eat it warm or at room temperature, on its own or with some good mayonnaise.

Serves 4

4 medium globe artichokes
4 lemons, halved
¾ cup dill, finely chopped
½ cup tarragon (leaves and stalks), finely chopped
½ cup parsley (leaves and stalks), finely chopped
1 onion, finely chopped
salt and black pepper
6 tbsp olive oil
1¾ cups green peas (fresh or frozen)
½ tsp sugar
1 garlic clove, crushed

Trim off the artichoke stalks close to the base, so that later they can sit flat in the pan. Tear off and discard the thick outer leaves, then use a small sharp knife to trim and tidy the base. Cut each artichoke vertically in half. Remove and discard the hairy choke and some of the internal purple leaves, to create a cavity in the heart of the artichoke. Rub all the cut surfaces immediately with the juice of one lemon and place in a bowl of cold water.

Mix the chopped herbs and onion with plenty of salt and pepper. Drain the artichokes and stuff the cavity in each half with the herb mix so that it is full but levelled. Keep the excess stuffing. Reshape each artichoke and use string to tie the halves back together closely.

Stand the four reconstructed artichokes in a saucepan just big enough to hold them close together. Add the juice of two lemons, the squeezed lemon halves and plenty of salt. Fill with water almost to cover the artichokes, leaving the top ¼ inch out of the water. Simmer on low heat for 20 to 35 minutes, making sure the artichoke bottoms are always immersed in water (keep the pan covered if the artichokes are not too big; otherwise top up with water during the cooking). To check if they are done, stick in a knife at the base. The artichoke heart should be soft throughout. Gently lift the artichokes from the pan and leave to drain for 5 minutes.

Meanwhile, sauté the remaining stuffing with 4 tablespoons of the olive oil for about 3 minutes. Add the peas, sugar, garlic and 5 tablespoons of the artichoke cooking liquid. Cook for 2 minutes more, then taste and add salt and pepper as needed. Add the juice of the remaining lemon (or more if you like).

Transfer the warm artichokes to serving plates and remove the string. Pile the lemony peas on top, drizzle generously with oil and serve.

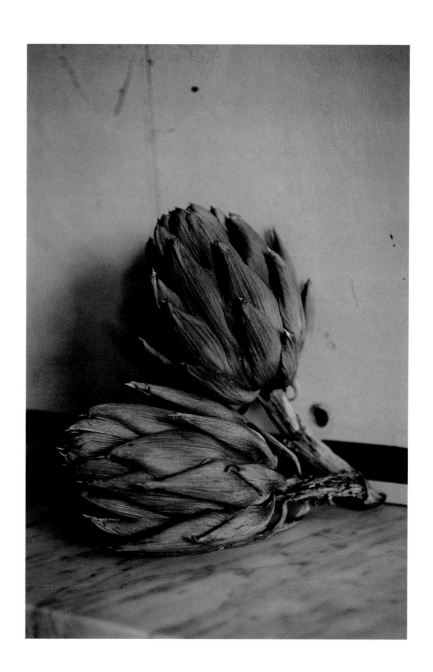

# Asparagus, fennel and beets with verjus

Verjus, or verjuice, is a sour juice made from unripe grapes. It was very popular in medieval times and is still used for making sauces in a few traditional French dishes. I was reminded of it by Ramael Scully, the former evening chef of Ottolenghi in Islington. Scully trained as a chef in Australia, where verjus has been regaining popularity in recent years as an alternative to vinegar in sauces and dressings, mainly thanks to the food writer Maggie Beer. Here, reduced verjus, with its sweetness and mild acidity, works wonders with raw vegetables.

Serves 4 as a starter
4 mini beets (about ¼ lb)
1⅓ cups verjus
4 tbsp grapeseed oil
salt and black pepper
4 to 5 oz fresh pencil-thin asparagus,
    or normal asparagus
½ large fennel bulb (¼ lb), halved
    vertically
¼ cup pine nuts, toasted
1 tbsp dill leaves to garnish

Preheat the oven to 400°F. Trim most of the stalk from the beets, leaving a little at the top of each beet for the look. Put them into an ovenproof dish, cover it with foil and bake for about 45 minutes, or until the beets are cooked through. Remove from the oven and leave to cool down before cutting into halves or quarters (you may want to peel them if the skin is tough).

Pour the verjus into a small saucepan, bring to a light simmer and leave it to reduce to about 3 tablespoons. Transfer to a mixing bowl and allow to cool down, then whisk in the grapeseed oil and salt and pepper to taste. Put aside.

If using normal asparagus, cut the spears on a sharp angle into long and very thin slices, or use a potato peeler to make "shavings." Place the fennel half cut-side down on a mandolin and shave into paper-thin slices. The slices will have a hand shape.

To assemble, arrange the vegetables on small serving plates. Scatter the pine nuts on top and drizzle over the dressing. Garnish with dill and serve.

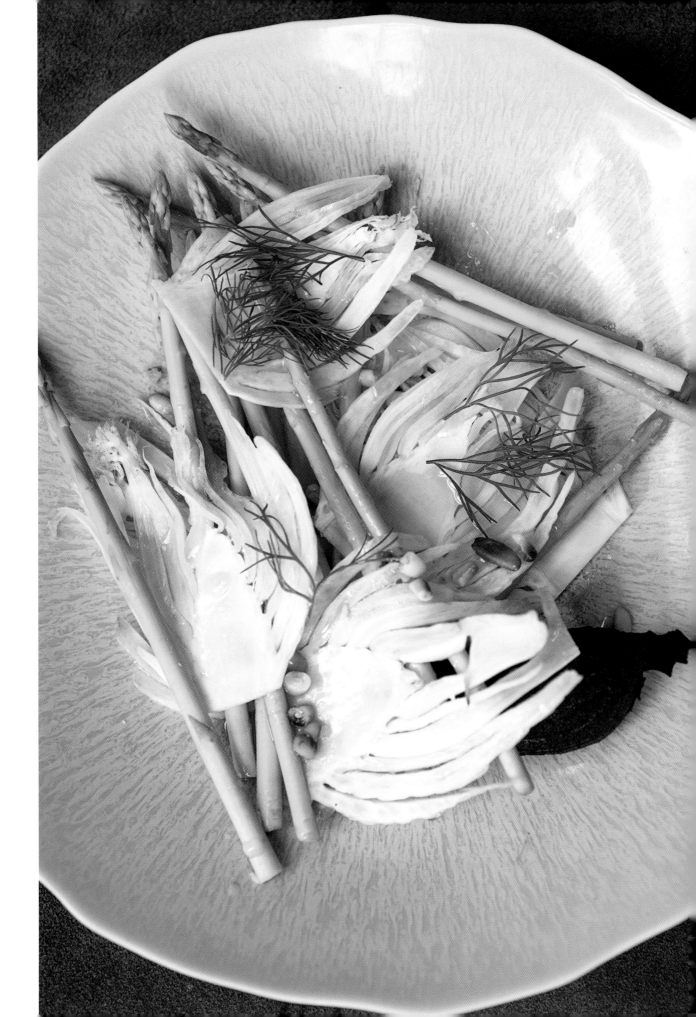

# Caramelized fennel with goat cheese

Goat's curd, a light cheese made from goat's milk, is known for its soft and creamy, yet not terribly unctuous, texture and for its wonderful freshness. It's hard to get, though. You'll want to ask around at your local farmers' market or a good cheese shop.

Still, there is no need to get despondent if you can't find it. There is an abundance of young and fresh goat cheeses that will do the trick equally well. My favorite is Caprini freschi, from Piedmont in Italy.

Serves 4
4 small fennel bulbs
3½ tbsp unsalted butter
3 tbsp olive oil, plus extra to finish
2 tbsp sugar
1 tsp fennel seeds
coarse sea salt and black pepper
1 garlic clove, crushed
¾ cup roughly chopped dill (leaves and stalks)
5 oz young and creamy goat cheese
grated zest of 1 lemon

Start by preparing the fennel bulbs. First take off the leafy fronds and keep them for the garnish. Then slice off some of the root part and remove any tough or brown outer layers, making sure the base still holds everything together. Cut each bulb lengthways into ½-inch-thick slices.

Melt half the butter with half the oil in a large frying pan placed over high heat. When the butter starts to foam add a layer of sliced fennel. Do not overcrowd the pan and don't turn the fennel over or stir it around in the pan until one side has become light golden, which will take about 2 minutes. Then turn the slices over using tongs and cook for a further 1 to 2 minutes. Remove from the pan. Continue with the rest of the fennel, using up the remaining butter and oil.

Once all the fennel has been seared, add the sugar, fennel seeds and plenty of salt and pepper to the pan. Fry for 30 seconds, then return all the fennel slices to the pan and caramelize them gently for 1 to 2 minutes (they need to remain firm inside so just allow them to be coated in the melting sugar and seeds). Remove the fennel from the pan and leave to cool down on a plate.

To serve, toss the fennel in a bowl with the garlic and dill. Taste and adjust the seasoning. Arrange on a serving plate and dot with spoonfuls of goat cheese. Finish with a drizzle of oil and a scattering of lemon zest. Garnish with the fennel fronds. Serve at room temperature.

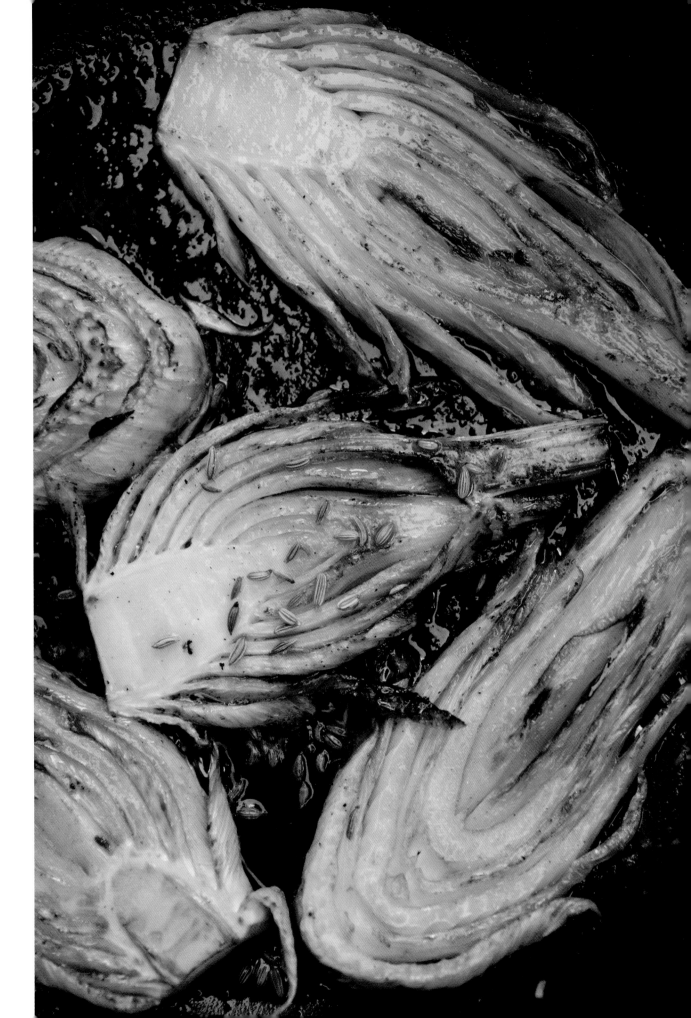

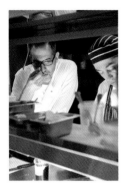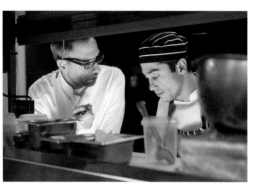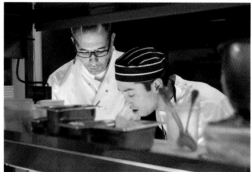

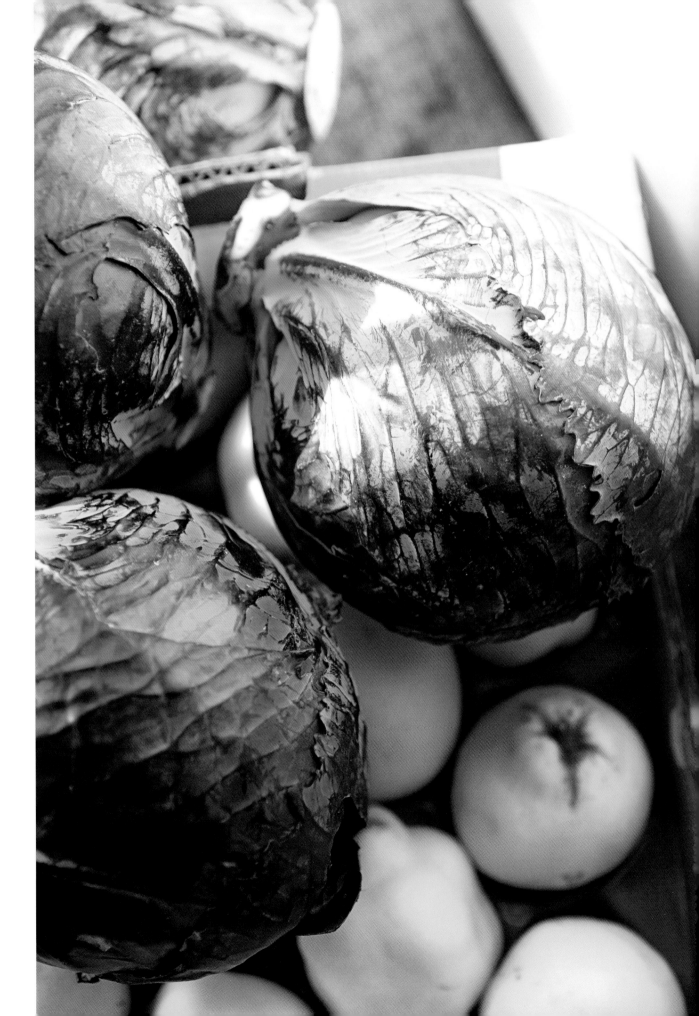

# Globe artichokes with crushed fava beans

My grandmother, Luciana Ottolenghi, formerly Cohen, who's had a huge influence on my taste buds and on my dad's cooking, was born to a Jewish family from Rome. In this recipe I pay homage to the way Roman Jews cook their artichokes, deep-frying them in olive oil, although I take it in a totally different direction.

Serves 2 as a starter
1¾ cups shelled fava beans (fresh or frozen)
1 small garlic clove, crushed
good-quality extra-virgin olive oil
1½ tsp Maldon sea salt
black pepper
2 to 3 globe artichokes, depending on size
juice of 3 lemons, plus 2 extra lemon halves to serve
1 egg, beaten
3 tbsp panko
3 tbsp chopped mint
2 tbsp chopped dill

Start with the fava beans. Bring a saucepan of water to the boil. Throw in the beans and blanch for 3 minutes. Drain, refresh under cold water and leave in the colander to dry. Once cool and dry, remove the outer skins of the beans by pressing each gently between your thumb and forefinger. Discard the skins.

Put the shelled beans into the bowl of a food processor. Add the garlic, 4 tablespoons olive oil, ½ teaspoon of the salt and some black pepper, and crush the beans roughly in a few pulses (you can also do this by hand using a fork). Make sure you don't process them into a purée. Set aside.

To prepare the artichokes, cut off most of the stalk and pull off the tough outer leaves. Once you reach the softer, pale leaves, take a sharp serrated knife and trim off the top so you are left with the base only. Scrape it clean with a little sharp knife, removing any remaining tough leaves and the hairy choke. You can now cut the resulting hearts in half or leave them whole. Rub them all over with the juice of one of the lemons and place in a bowl of cold water. Add the juice of another lemon and all the squeezed lemon halves.

Bring a medium saucepan of water to the boil. Carefully drop in the artichoke hearts and simmer for 7 to 10 minutes, or until a knife will pierce them easily. Drain well and dry on a dish towel. Place the artichoke hearts in a bowl with the beaten egg and mix well. Spread the panko on a plate and season with 1 teaspoon salt. Lift the artichokes from the bowl with a fork and into the panko. Coat them in the crumbs.

Pour enough olive oil into a small saucepan to come 1¼ inches up the sides and heat up until almost smoking. Add a couple of artichokes at a time to the hot oil and fry for about 4 minutes, or until golden, turning them to color evenly. Transfer to a plate lined with paper towels and sprinkle with a little salt.

Stir the chopped herbs and the juice of the third lemon into the crushed beans. Spoon some over each serving plate. Place one or two artichoke pieces on top and spoon more crushed beans on top or around. Finish with a drizzle of olive oil and serve with a lemon half.

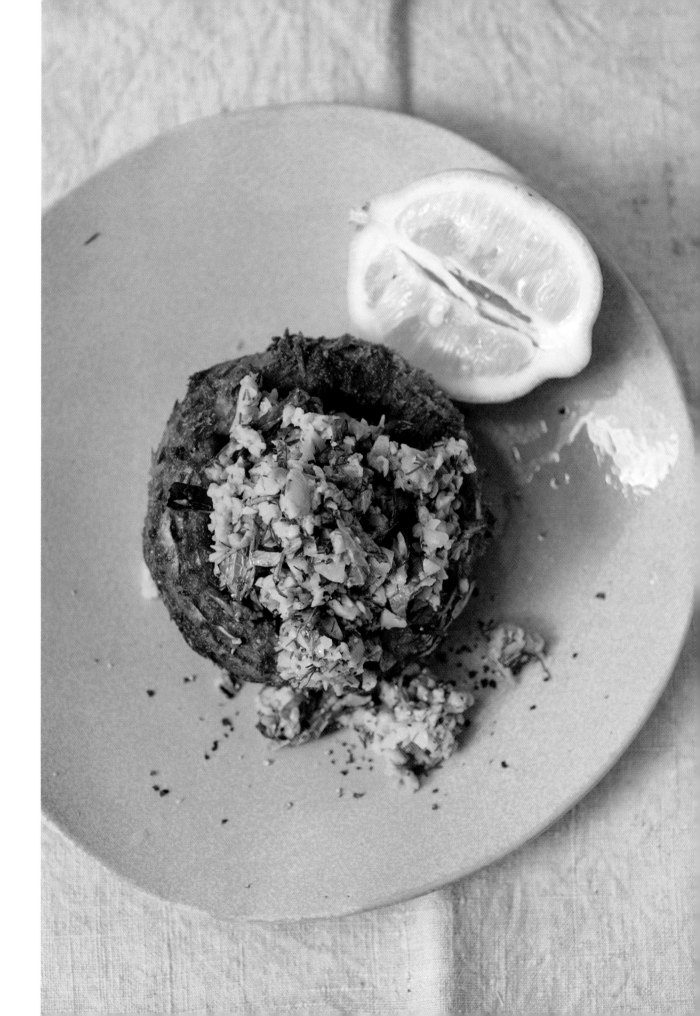

# Artichoke gratin

I am all for frozen vegetables, especially when used for hearty, long-cooked dishes like this one. Here, in particular, you'll save yourself tons of work if you can get a couple of bags of frozen artichoke hearts, without sacrificing much flavor. Serve the gratin with Lettuce Salad (page 146).

Serves 4–6

1¾ lbs frozen artichoke hearts, thawed, or about 20 medium-sized globe artichokes

grated zest and juice of 4 large lemons

2 medium onions, thinly sliced

¼ cup olive oil

salt and black pepper

3 tbsp chopped thyme

6 tbsp chopped parsley

**Béchamel**

4 tbsp unsalted butter

⅓ cup plus 1 tbsp all-purpose flour

1 cup water

1 cup milk

¾ tsp salt

¾ cup ricotta

6 tbsp grated Parmesan

If using fresh artichokes, prepare them first. Use your hands to pull off the hard outer leaves until you reach the center with its small softer leaves. Rub about one-third of the lemon juice on the artichokes as you clean them. Use a small, sharp serrated knife to trim off all the leaves, then scrape away the hairy choke from the center. Discard the leaves and choke.

Cut the artichoke hearts (freshly prepared or frozen) into ¼-inch-thick slices. Put at once into a pot with plenty of water and all the lemon juice (you may have used some already when cleaning the fresh artichokes; add whatever is left). Bring to the boil and simmer for about 5 minutes, or until the artichokes are tender (the frozen ones won't take as long as the fresh). Drain.

While the artichokes are cooking, put the onions in a pan with the olive oil and some salt and pepper. Cook on medium heat for about 10 minutes, or until golden, stirring occasionally. Add the onions and oil to the cooked artichokes together with the lemon zest, thyme and parsley. Stir gently to mix. Taste and add more salt and pepper, if you like. Set aside.

Preheat the oven to 375°F.

To make the béchamel. Melt the butter in a small saucepan. Add the flour and cook on medium heat, stirring all the time, for about 2 minutes. Make sure the mix doesn't brown much. Mix the water and milk and slowly add to the saucepan as you whisk. Add the salt and keep on cooking and whisking on low heat for about 10 minutes, or until the sauce is thick and creamy.

Gently mix together the artichokes and béchamel, then pour into a small ovenproof dish that's been lightly greased with oil. Make small holes in the artichoke mix and into each drop about 1 teaspoonful of ricotta. Cover the dish with foil and bake for 30 minutes.

Remove the foil and scatter the Parmesan over the top. Increase the oven temperature to 400°F. Continue baking for 15 to 20 minutes, or until the Parmesan turns golden brown and the béchamel is bubbling away. Remove from the oven and serve hot or warm.

# Okra with tomato, lemon and cilantro

Here's a secret ingredient I pick up from the freezer of a Lebanese market in London: tiny Egyptian okra, perfectly firm, packed with flavor. Almost as important, it comes already trimmed.

Serves 4

4 tbsp olive oil

1½ tsp coriander seeds

1 medium onion, thinly sliced

2 red bell peppers, cut into ⅜-inch-wide strips

1 mild fresh red chile, seeded and chopped

¾ cup chopped parsley leaves

¾ cup chopped cilantro leaves

2 large tomatoes, chopped (or 1¾ cups canned)

¾ cup water

1 tsp sweet paprika

2 tsp sugar

salt

4 cups okra (fresh or frozen)

3 tbsp finely chopped skin of preserved lemon

30 pitted black olives, each cut in half

1½ tbsp lemon juice

1 tbsp shredded mint

Preheat the oven to 400°F. Heat up 2 tablespoons of the oil in a large saucepan. Add the coriander seeds and onion and sauté on medium heat for 10 minutes, or until the onion softens without coloring. Add the red peppers, chile, parsley and half the chopped cilantro. Cook and stir for a further 5 minutes.

Next, add the tomatoes, water, paprika, sugar and salt to taste. Leave to simmer, covered, for 15 minutes. Remove the lid and continue cooking for about 5 minutes, or until the sauce is thick and has lost most of the excess liquid.

While making the tomato sauce, prepare the okra (in case you couldn't get any of the prepared frozen variety). Take a small pointy knife and carefully remove the stem end; try not to cut very low, keeping the end of the stem to seal the main body of the fruit so the seeds are not exposed. Mix the okra with the remaining 2 tablespoons of oil and some salt and spread over a roasting pan. Roast for 15 to 20 minutes, or until just tender but still firm.

Add the cooked okra to the tomato sauce. Stir gently, also mixing in the preserved lemon, olives and half of the remaining chopped cilantro. Taste and adjust the seasoning.

You can serve the dish warm with steamed bulgur wheat or couscous, or leave to cool down and serve at room temperature with bread and other mezze. In both cases, mix in the lemon juice just before serving and garnish with the remaining cilantro and the mint.

# Green gazpacho

There are a million recipes around for gazpacho, which is by far my favorite cold soup. This one, a green variation, is loosely based on *tarator*, a cold yogurt and cucumber soup from the Balkans. A proper freestanding blender works best here but an immersion blender could also be used.

Serves 6

**Croutons**
2 thick slices sourdough bread
4 tbsp olive oil
salt

2 celery stalks (including the leaves)
2 small green bell peppers, seeded
6 mini cucumbers (1¼ lbs), peeled
3 slices stale white bread, crusts removed
1 fresh green chile (or less if you don't want it too hot)
4 garlic cloves
1 tsp sugar
1½ cups walnuts, lightly toasted
6 cups baby spinach
1 cup basil leaves
2 tbsp chopped parsley
4 tbsp sherry vinegar
1 cup olive oil
3 tbsp Greek yogurt
about 2 cups water
9 oz ice cubes
2 tsp salt
white pepper

To make the croutons. Preheat the oven to 375°F. Cut the bread into ¾-inch cubes and toss them with the oil and a bit of salt. Spread on a baking sheet and bake for about 10 minutes, or until the croutons turn golden and crisp. Remove from the oven and allow to cool down.

Roughly chop the celery, bell peppers, cucumbers, bread, chile and garlic. Place in a blender and add the sugar, walnuts, spinach, basil, parsley, vinegar, oil, yogurt, most of the water, half the ice cubes, the salt and some white pepper. Blitz the soup until smooth. Add more water, if needed, to get your preferred consistency. Taste the soup and adjust the seasoning.

Lastly, add the remaining ice and pulse once or twice, just to crush it a little. Serve at once, with the croutons.

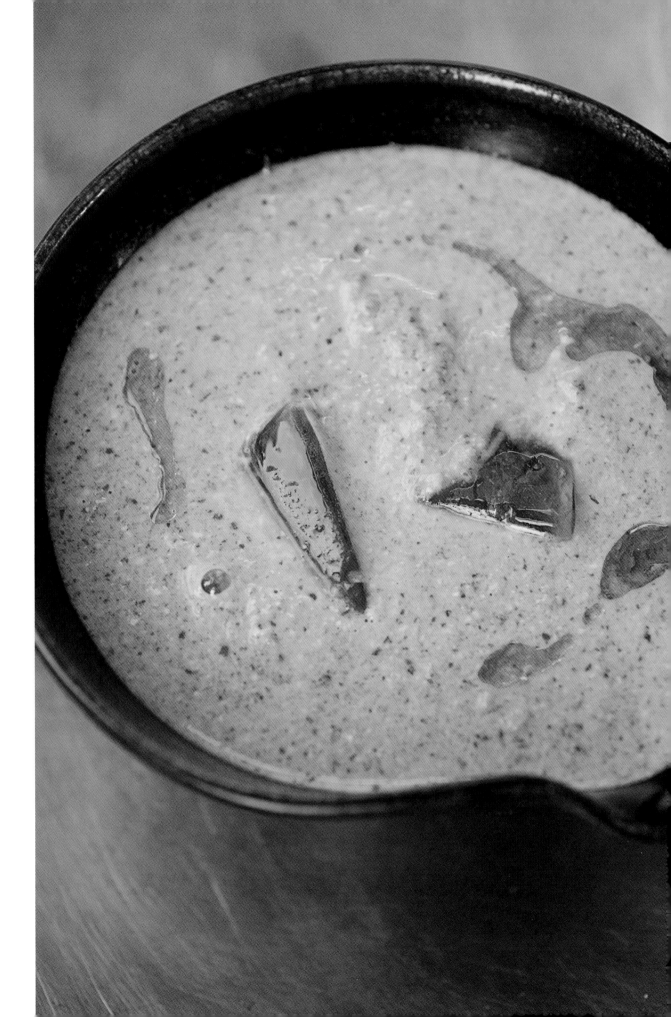

# Asparagus mimosa

This traditional way with asparagus is probably my favorite. It is simple and therefore relies on the quality of the asparagus itself more than anything else. See if you can get the spears from a farmers' market or the shop at a farm where they have been freshly picked. Roughly chopped tarragon sprinkled on top will make a good addition.

Serves 4 as a starter
2 eggs
2 bunches of medium asparagus
2 tbsp good-quality olive oil
2 tsp small capers, drained
1 tsp Maldon sea salt
black pepper

Gently place your eggs in a saucepan of boiling water and simmer for 9 minutes. Remove the eggs from the pan and immerse them in a large bowl of cold water. After a few minutes, take them out of the water and leave to cool down completely. Peel the eggs and grate them on a coarse cheese grater.

Bend the asparagus until the tough bottom ends snap off; discard the ends. Place the spears in a large pot of boiling water and cook for 3 minutes, or until tender. It may take slightly longer if they are thick.

Drain and, while still warm but not hot, divide among four serving plates. Drizzle the oil over the asparagus and sprinkle with the capers, salt and some pepper. Top with the grated egg, staying close to the center of the stalks so that the tips and bases remain visible.

# Char-grilled asparagus

Here asparagus spears are simply cooked on a ridged griddle pan. The fact that they are not boiled means that they keep more of their original flavor. The texture, though, is slightly more sinewy than when boiling or steaming. I suggest using a mild feta, not too salty, or another type of mild sheep's cheese from the Balkans (see Dates and Turkish Sheep's Cheese, page 280). Serve warm, as a starter, or as part of a mezze spread.

Serves 4
2 bunches of asparagus
2 tbsp grapeseed oil, plus extra to finish
1 tsp Maldon sea salt
black pepper
8 thin slices good-quality feta (2½ oz in total), or a few spoonfuls of ricotta
grated zest of 1 lemon

Snap off the tough ends of the asparagus and discard. Toss the spears in the grapeseed oil and sprinkle with the salt and some pepper. Lay the asparagus in a hot griddle pan, placing them perpendicular to the ridges of the pan. Cook for 6 to 9 minutes, turning occasionally, or until just al dente and lightly charred.

Arrange the asparagus on four serving plates. Add the slices of feta and drizzle some grapeseed oil on top and around the plate. Finish with the lemon zest and a bit of black pepper.

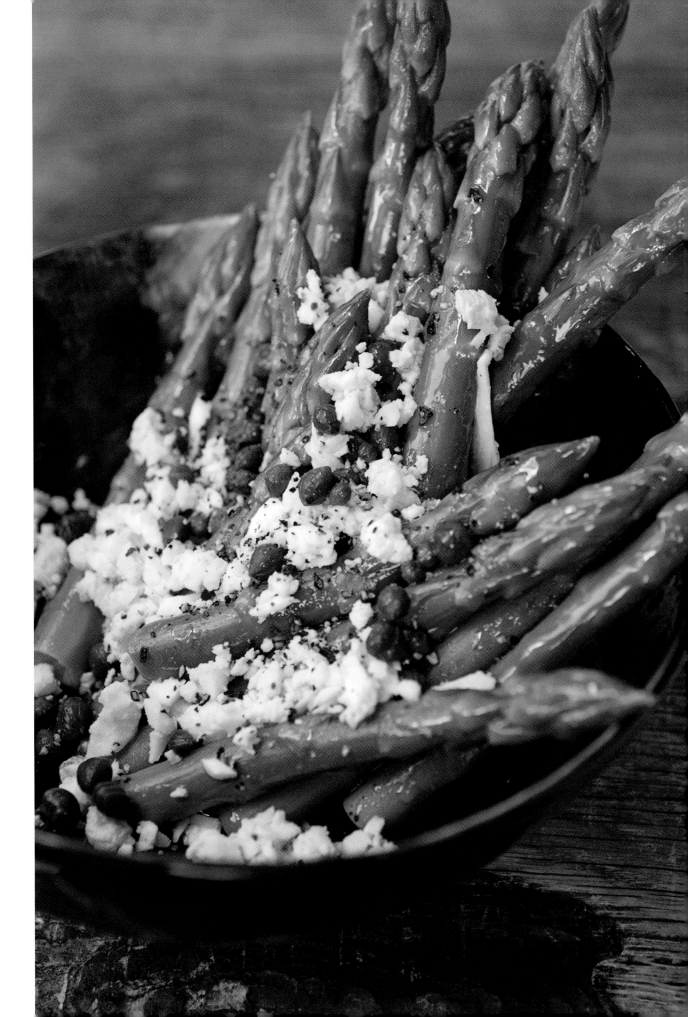

# Asparagus vichyssoise

My love for cold soups comes from my parents. When I was a child my mother used to make the most refreshing gazpacho for us, to alleviate the dry heat of the Jerusalem summer. It was marvelous – a little sweet, a little sour and totally light. When I recently shut myself up at my parents' house, to finally get on with all the recipe intros for this book, my father made one of his glorious creations: a cold creamy soup of potato, freshly picked basil, cucumber chunks and loads of goat's milk yogurt from the neighboring goat farm. I am afraid I can't replicate this in London.

The ideal time for making *my* cold soup is toward the end of the asparagus season, in the early summer, when the spears are often thick and woody and not good enough to eat as they are. Serve with crusty bread dipped in olive oil.

Serves 4
1 medium potato
2 medium leeks
1 lb asparagus
1½ tbsp unsalted butter
2½ cups good-quality vegetable stock
1 tsp sugar
salt and white pepper
3 tbsp heavy cream
6 tbsp Greek yogurt
grated zest of ½ lemon

Peel the potato and dice roughly. Chop off and discard the tough green ends of the leeks. Cut through the pale center, then wash and slice roughly. Trim off and discard the woody base of the asparagus. Cut all but three of the spears into ¾-inch pieces, keeping the tips separate. Reserve whole spears.

Place the vegetables, except for the asparagus tips, with the butter in a medium saucepan and sauté on medium heat for about 4 minutes; make sure they don't take on any color. Cover the vegetables with the stock and add the sugar and some salt and white pepper. Bring to a boil, then simmer, covered, for 40 minutes. At the end of this time add the asparagus tips and continue cooking for 10 minutes.

Once done, blitz the soup well in a blender until very smooth. Gently fold in the cream and half the yogurt. Allow the soup to come to room temperature, then chill.

While the soup is cooling down, bring a pan of water to the boil and blanch the reserved asparagus for 2 minutes; drain and refresh under plenty of cold water. Shred.

Pour the cold soup into bowls. Spoon a dollop of yogurt on top of each and swirl with the tip of a skewer. Place the shredded asparagus in the center and garnish with lemon zest.

# Mee goreng

All over Malaysia a profusion of street food is served in big open-air complexes. The different stalls prepare cheap, cheerful and incredibly delicious dishes from Malay, Chinese or Indian cuisines. Since everything is so tempting you often end up with a table still piled with delicacies and no stomach capacity. The attraction of this type of dining is that it is both fresh and complex. Many dishes are prepared from raw in front of your eyes, using great ingredients, which makes it far superior to many Western solutions for fast food. I was guided through a recent Malaysian adventure by Helen Goh and her affectionate family, the Lees, who have taught me many culinary secrets.

This Malay dish (pictured on pages 186 to 187) takes only a few minutes to make (once you have a little bit of prep out of the way) and is unique in its many layers and depth of flavors. If you want to serve more than two people you'll need to start again with a second batch, because double quantities will be too much for one wok.

Serves 2

2 tbsp peanut oil

½ onion, diced

8 oz firm tofu, cut into ⅜-inch-thick
    strips

4 oz green beans, trimmed and cut in
    half at an angle

4 oz choi sum (or bok choy), cut into
    large chunks (both leaves and stalks)

11 oz fresh egg noodles

1½ tsp ground coriander

1 tsp ground cumin

2 tsp sambal oelek (or another savory
    chile paste), plus extra to serve

2 tsp thick soy sauce

2 tsp light soy sauce

1 tbsp water

2 oz Mung bean sprouts

handful of shredded iceberg lettuce

1 tbsp crisp-fried shallots

lemon wedges to serve

Set a wok or a large pan on high heat. Once hot, add the oil and then the onion, and cook for about 1 minute to soften a bit. Add the tofu and French beans and cook for 2 to 3 minutes to give the tofu a bit of color. Stir gently as you cook, trying not to break up the tofu.

Next, add the choi sum. When it wilts add the noodles and carefully spread them in the wok using tongs or large chopsticks. You want the noodles to get a lot of heat, almost to fry. Mix gently, cooking the noodles for about 2 minutes. Now add the spices, sambal oelek, soy sauces, water and bean sprouts and toss carefully. Cook for about a minute, or until the noodles are semisoft.

When ready, top with lettuce, transfer to serving bowls and sprinkle with crisp shallots. On the side, serve lemon wedges and a small bowl of extra sambal olek.

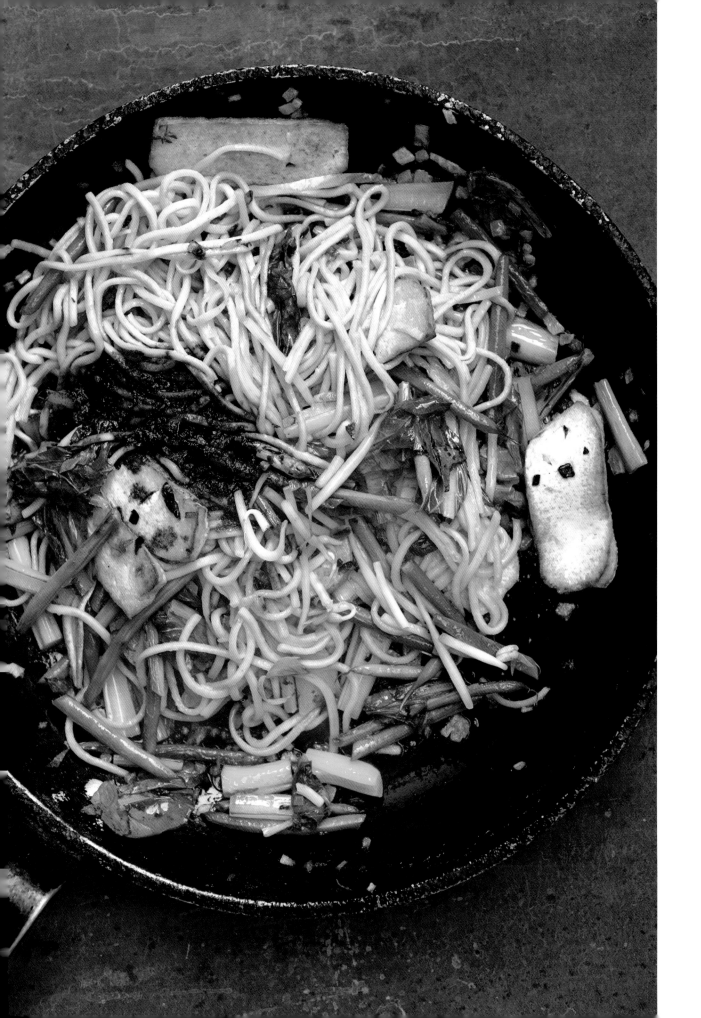

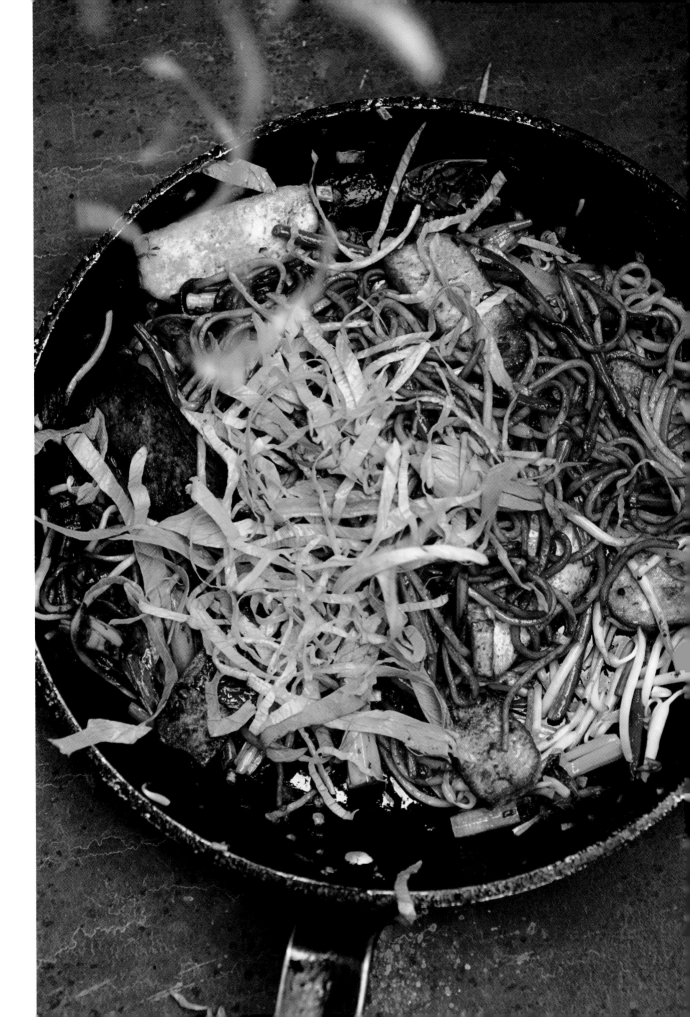

# Soba noodles with wakame

In 2009 I travelled to Tokyo with the sole purpose of eating. I have always liked Japanese food but this time I was blown away, completely taken over by food and by the fact that the Japanese, like no other culture that I know of, are *all* foodies. It was fantastic being in the company of so many who, just like me, are willing to line up for the best sponge cake in the world, the finest slice of raw fish or the greatest soba noodles. The latter I tasted, along with dozens of businessmen in fancy suits, at Yabusoba, an unassuming restaurant in the old neighborhood of Kanda.

Soba noodles, made of buckwheat, are often served cold with a flavorful dipping sauce. Wakame is a sea vegetable with a mild salty flavor and a slurpy texture. Other varieties of seaweed can be used as substitutes here. Or, if ocean flavor is not your thing, replace with thinly sliced radishes.

Serves 4–6
2 large cucumbers (skin on)
2 tsp salt
11 oz soba noodles
one 2-oz package wakame

Sauce
2 tbsp rice vinegar
grated zest of 2 limes
¼ cup lime juice
1 tbsp grated fresh ginger
2 fresh red chiles, finely chopped (or
     less if you don't like it too hot)
1 tbsp palm sugar
2 tbsp toasted sesame oil
2 tbsp peanut oil
1 tbsp sweet chile sauce
1 garlic clove, crushed
¾ tsp salt

½ cup toasted sesame seeds
2 cups cilantro leaves, roughly chopped
¾ cup mint leaves, roughly chopped
1⅓ cups radish sprouts, plus extra to
     garnish

Shred the cucumbers using a mandolin or the shredding blade in a food processor. Place the thin strips in a colander, sprinkle with the salt and stir well, then leave to drain for at least 30 minutes.

Put the noodles in a pan of boiling water and cook for 4 to 5 minutes, or as instructed on the packet. Drain and rinse in a stream of cold water to stop the cooking. Leave to dry.

Soak the wakame in warm water for about 10 minutes, or until it softens up; drain. Remove the tough "stalks" and discard. Cut or tear the rest into large pieces and put into a large mixing bowl. Add the cooked noodles and cucumber to the wakame.

To make the sauce. Whisk together all of the sauce ingredients.

Add to the noodle mix. Stir gently, then add the sesame seeds, cilantro, mint and sprouts. Stir well again and taste – you want a sweetish tart flavor with a kick. If needed, add more salt, vinegar or sugar.

To serve, pile the noodles in serving bowls and garnish with radish sprouts.

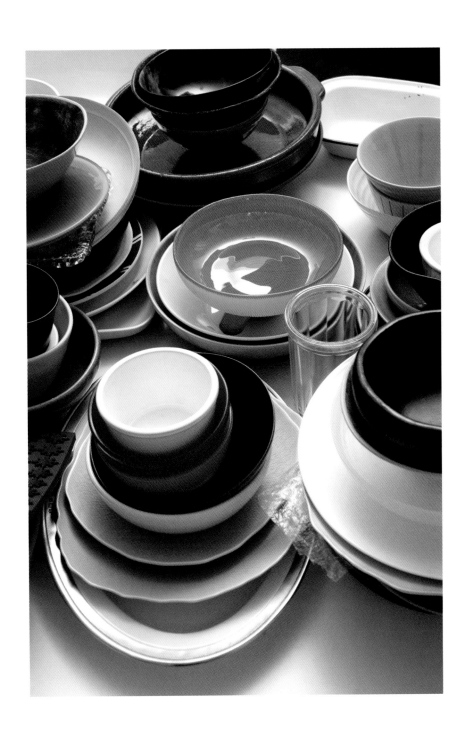

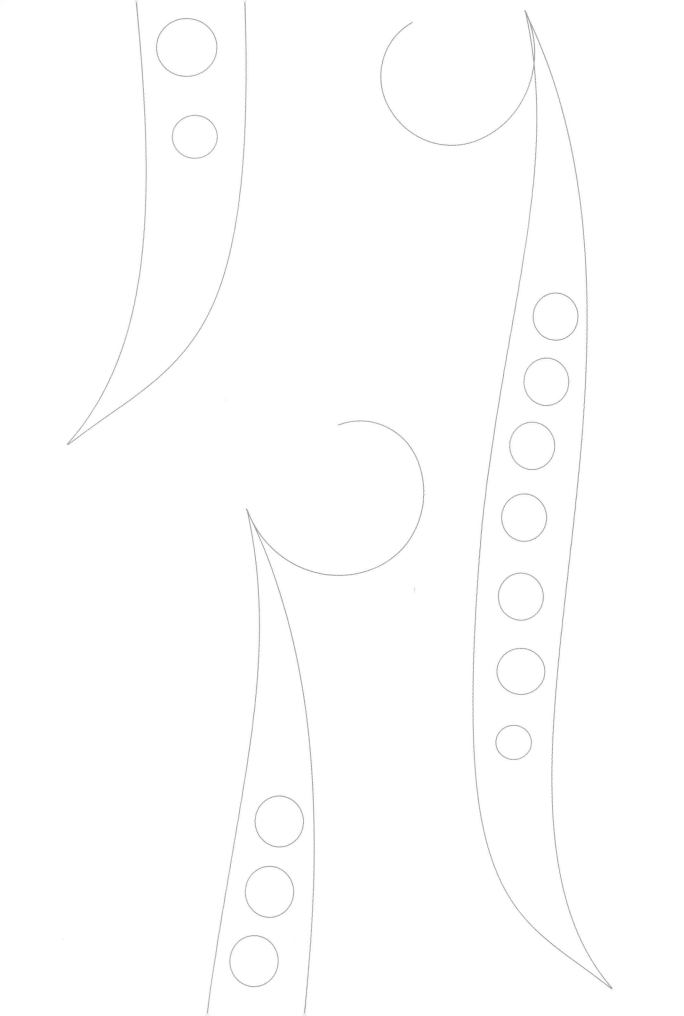

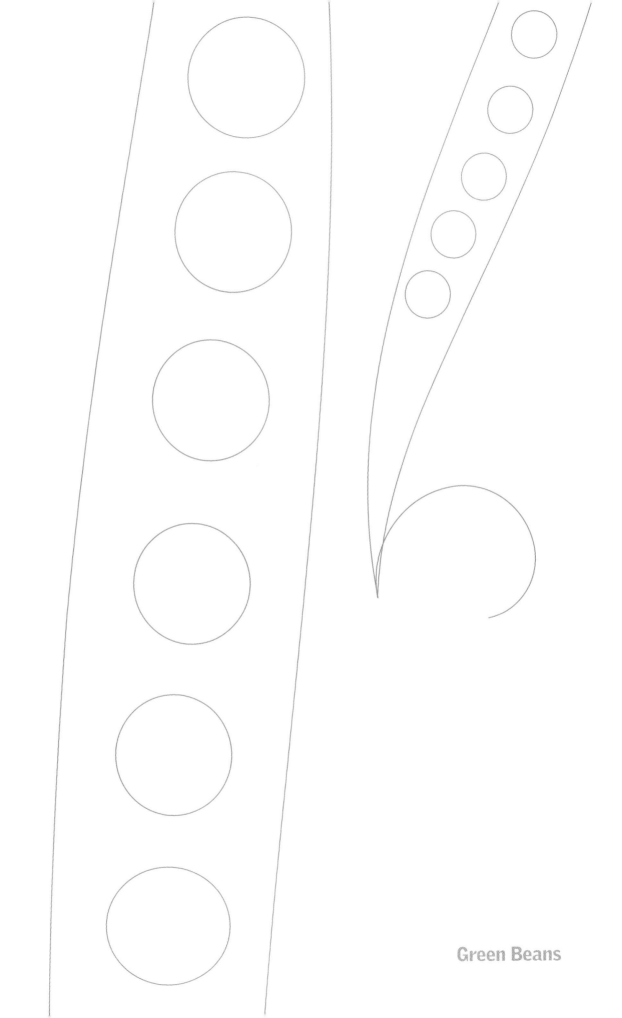

Green Beans

# Mixed beans with many spices and lovage

This is a wonderfully aromatic dish that uses an abundance of spices, resulting in a curry-like delicacy. It can be served warm with a mix of basmati and wild rice or at room temperature as a side dish.

Lovage looks like flat-leaf parsley but tastes like intense celery. Use it sparingly and you'll find it adds tons of character to salads, lentil dishes and creamy sauces. If you can't get hold of it, substitute with cilantro or tarragon.

Serves 4
3 tbsp olive oil
1 medium onion, finely chopped
2 garlic cloves, chopped
2 tsp tomato paste
½ tsp ground cumin
½ tsp ground turmeric
½ tsp ground coriander
1 tsp ground ginger
1 tsp ground cardamom
pinch of ground cloves
salt and black pepper
one 14-oz can chopped tomatoes (with
    their juices)
1 tsp sugar
1½ cups sugar snap peas, halved at an
    angle
1 cup large string beans, sliced at an
    angle
1¾ cups shelled fava beans (fresh or
    frozen)
2 tbsp chopped lovage

Heat up the oil in a large pan and add the onion. Sauté on medium heat for 3 minutes, stirring frequently; add the garlic and cook for 1 more minute. Now add the tomato paste, spices and some salt and pepper and keep on cooking and stirring for another minute.

Next, add the tomatoes, sugar and all the peas and beans. Stir to mix. Bring to the boil, then cover and simmer gently for 15 to 20 minutes, or until the sugar snaps are cooked through but are still crunchy. Taste and add salt and pepper as you like. Stir in the lovage just before serving warm or cooled.

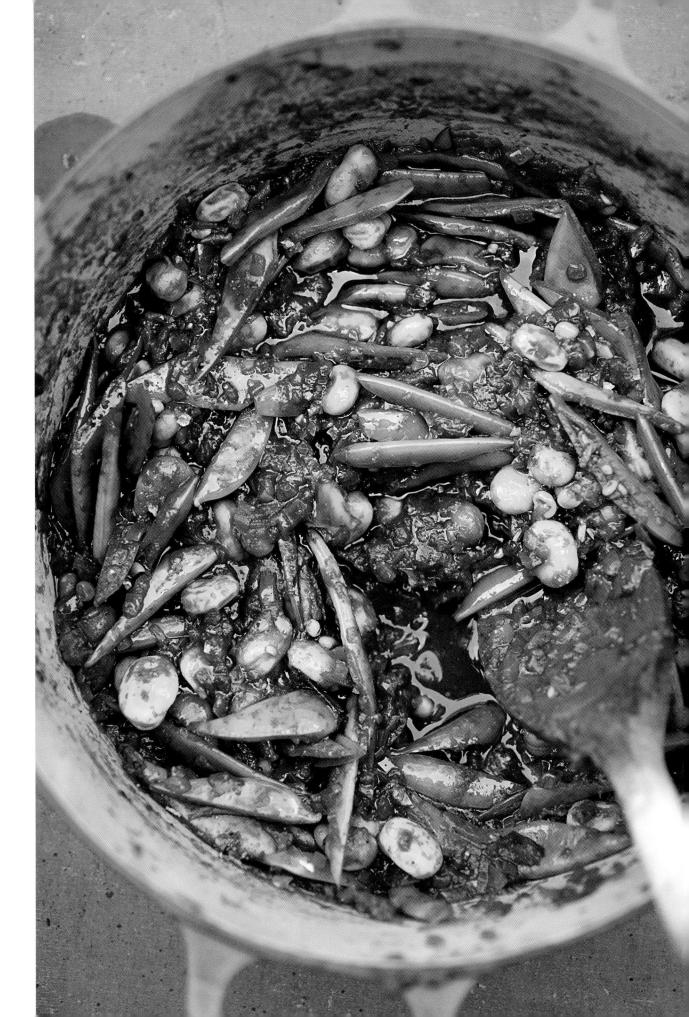

# Fava bean burgers

When this recipe first appeared in the *Guardian* I didn't mention skinning the fava beans. This time I have done so because I decided to make the burgers smoother and more refined. I have to admit that the skinning does add a fair amount of work, probably 30 minutes, but I believe the upgrade is worth it. I did save some time, though, by leaving out a sour cream and lemon sauce from the original. If you insist, serve with the condiment for the Sweet Potato Cakes on page 32.

Serves 4

¾ tsp cumin seeds

¾ tsp coriander seeds

¾ tsp fennel seeds

½ lb (about 6 cups) spinach

3 tbsp olive oil

1 lb (about 3 cups) shelled fava beans
(fresh or frozen)

¾ lb potatoes, peeled and roughly diced

½ fresh green chile, seeded and finely
chopped

2 garlic cloves, crushed

¼ tsp ground turmeric

salt and black pepper

3 tbsp chopped cilantro

6 tbsp dried breadcrumbs

1 egg

½ cup sunflower oil

4 lemon wedges

Put the whole seeds in a pan and dry-roast over high heat for 3 to 4 minutes, or until they start releasing their aromas. Grind to a powder in a mortar and pestle and leave aside.

Wilt the spinach in a hot pan with 1 tablespoon of the olive oil. When cool enough to handle, squeeze out any liquid, then chop roughly and set aside.

Blanch the fava beans in boiling water for about a minute; drain and refresh under cold running water. Once cool enough to handle, remove and discard the skins (see page 202).

Cook the potatoes in boiling water for about 15 minutes, or until tender. Drain and tip into a large mixing bowl. Immediately add the skinned fava beans, crushed seeds, chile, garlic, turmeric, remaining 2 tablespoons of olive oil and some salt and pepper. Use a potato masher to mash it all up roughly; don't worry if some beans are not totally crushed. Next, add the wilted spinach, chopped cilantro and breadcrumbs. Taste to check the seasoning. Lastly, mix in the egg.

Wet your hands and shape the mix into fat patties that are roughly 2 inches in diameter and ¾ inch thick. Chill them for at least half an hour.

To cook, heat up the sunflower oil and fry the burgers on high heat for 5 minutes on each side, or until golden brown. Serve warm, with the lemon wedges.

# Gado-gado

Gado-gado is best described as a very substantial salad. You don't need anything else with it. A visit to an Asian grocer is essential for getting all the right ingredients, but some creative substitutes would probably also work. The satay sauce is a little work but it's worth every bit of the effort. Use it for marinating white meat or tofu, or just spoon over hot rice or rice noodles.

Serves 4

**Satay sauce**

4 garlic cloves, peeled

1 lemongrass stalk, roughly chopped

2½ tbsp sambal oelek (Indonesian crushed chile paste)

2 small pieces of galangal (or peeled fresh ginger)

4 medium shallots, peeled

⅓ cup vegetable oil

¾ tbsp salt

7 tbsp sugar

½ tbsp sweet paprika

2 tbsp thick tamarind water (tamarind pulp whisked with a little water and strained)

1½ cups roasted unsalted peanuts

1¾ cups water

1 cup coconut milk

1 tsp ground turmeric

2 medium potatoes, peeled and cut into wedges

½ medium cabbage, cut into chunks

1 cup bean sprouts

½ cup green beans, trimmed

½ medium cucumber, thickly sliced

4 hard-boiled eggs, quartered

4 oz firm tofu, cut into ⅜-inch-thick slices

cassava chips (or something else crunchy like deep-fried croutons or wonton skins)

3 tbsp cilantro leaves

crisp-fried shallots

To make the satay sauce. Use a small food processor to blitz the garlic, lemongrass, sambal oelek, galangal and shallots into a homogenous paste. Add a little bit of the vegetable oil, if needed, to bring everything together.

Heat up the remaining oil in a medium saucepan. Add the paste and cook on a gentle heat for 40 to 50 minutes, or until the oil starts separating from the paste. Stir regularly. Once ready, combine the salt, sugar and paprika and add to the spice paste. Also add the tamarind water. Cook for 10 minutes more.

While the paste is cooking, take the peanuts and crush them roughly in a food processor; they should be chunkier than ground almonds. Put the peanuts and water into a small saucepan and simmer on low heat for 20 to 25 minutes, or until the mixture thickens and most of the water has evaporated. Add the peanuts (plus water) to the cooked spice paste, stir in the coconut milk and there's your satay sauce. Keep it somewhere warm.

Have ready two pots of boiling water; add the turmeric to one of them. Cook the potatoes in the turmeric water until tender, then drain. In the other pot blanch the cabbage for 1 minute; remove, and blanch the bean sprouts for 30 seconds. Remove those, then blanch the green beans for 4 minutes and drain (no need to refresh). Keep these vegetables warm.

Take a large communal serving plate and pile up all the vegetables, eggs, tofu and most of the chips. Generously spoon warm satay sauce on top (you'll probably have a fair bit left over; you can keep it in the fridge for a few days), then sprinkle with the remaining chips, the cilantro and crisp shallots if you like. Serve warmish.

# Green bean salad with mustard seeds and tarragon

This salad – offering a good balance of clean freshness from the beans with the punchy complexity of the herbs and spices – works in plenty of contexts. Try it next to Two-Potato Vindaloo (page 18), along with Fried Lima Beans with Feta, Sorrel and Sumac (page 214), or as a side dish with grilled lamb chops.

Serves 4

1¼ cups green beans, trimmed

2¼ cups snow peas, trimmed

1¾ cups green peas (fresh or frozen)

2 tsp coriander seeds, roughly crushed with a mortar and pestle

1 tsp mustard seeds

3 tbsp olive oil

1 tsp nigella seeds

½ small red onion, finely chopped

1 mild fresh red chile, seeded and finely diced

1 garlic clove, crushed

grated zest of 1 lemon

2 tbsp chopped tarragon

coarse sea salt

1 cup baby chard leaves (optional)

Fill a medium saucepan with cold water and bring to the boil. Blanch the green beans for 4 minutes, then immediately lift them out of the pan and into iced water to refresh. Drain and dry.

Bring a fresh pan of water to the boil and blanch the snow peas for 1 minute only. Refresh, drain and dry. Use the same boiling water to blanch the peas for 20 seconds. Refresh, drain and dry. Combine the beans, snow peas and peas in a large mixing bowl.

Put the coriander seeds, mustard seeds and oil in a small saucepan and heat up. When the seeds begin to pop, pour the contents of the pan over the beans and peas. Toss together, then add the nigella seeds, red onion, chile, garlic, lemon zest and tarragon. Mix well and season with salt to taste.

Just before serving, gently fold the chard leaves, if using, in with the beans and peas, and spoon the salad onto plates or into bowls.

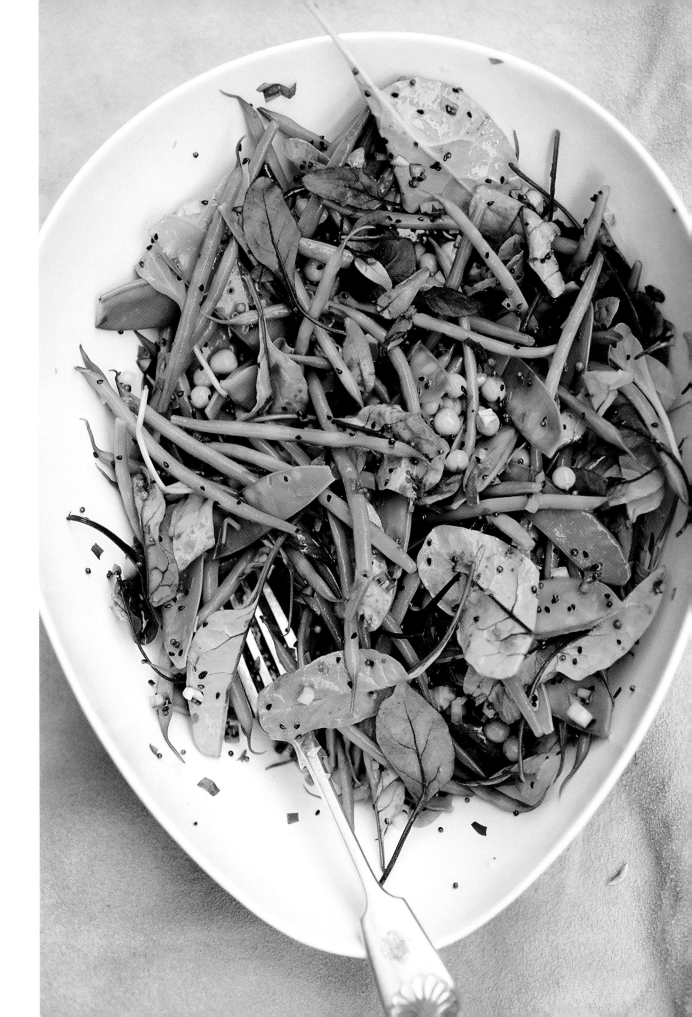

# Warm glass noodles and edamame

Until recently edamame, which are similar to fava beans but harder and nuttier, were only available in Japanese restaurants. Now, with their health benefits celebrated everywhere (they are full of protein, omega-3 fatty acids, vitamin A and more), these young soybeans are widely available, whether frozen and shelled, cooked or raw.

Edamame fit well in most salads and in warm dishes. This one makes a refreshing light meal. You can upgrade it by adding fried tofu and/or roasted peanuts.

Serves 4
7 oz glass (cellophane) noodles

Sauce
2 tbsp grated galangal or fresh ginger
juice of 4 limes
3 tbsp peanut oil
2 tbsp palm sugar
2 tsp seedless tamarind pulp or paste
1 tsp tamari
1 tsp fine sea salt

2 tbsp sunflower oil
3 garlic cloves, crushed
2½ cups shelled cooked edamame
3 green onions, thinly sliced (including the green parts)
1 fresh red chile, finely chopped
3 tbsp chopped cilantro, plus a few whole leaves to garnish
3 tbsp shredded fresh mint
3 tbsp sesame seeds, toasted
salt (optional)

Soak the noodles in a bowl of hot water for about 5 minutes, or until soft (don't leave them in the water for too long or they will get soggy). Drain and leave to dry.

To make the sauce. In a small bowl whisk together all of the sauce ingredients and set aside.

Heat the sunflower oil in a large frying pan or a wok and add the garlic. When it starts to turn golden, remove the pan from the heat and add the sauce and noodles. Gently stir together, then add most of the edamame and the green onions, chile, cilantro and mint. Stir everything together while you return the pan to the heat for a few seconds, just to warm through. Taste and season with salt, if you like.

Pile up on a large platter or in a shallow bowl and scatter over the remaining edamame and the sesame seeds. Garnish with cilantro leaves and serve. You can also serve this dish at room temperature, adjusting the seasoning when it is cool.

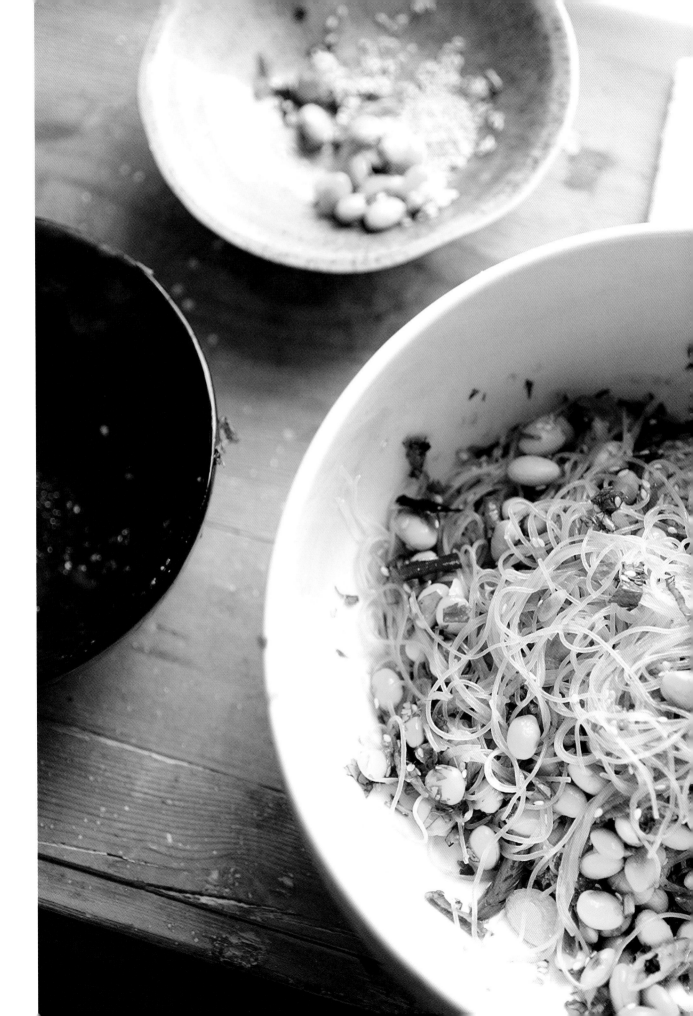

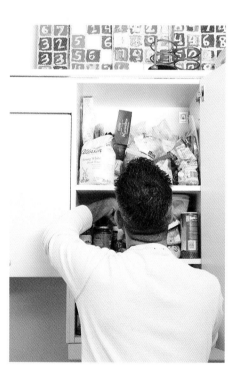

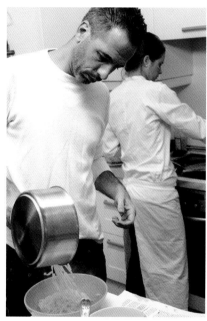

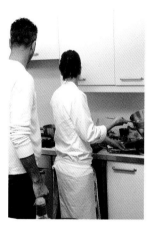

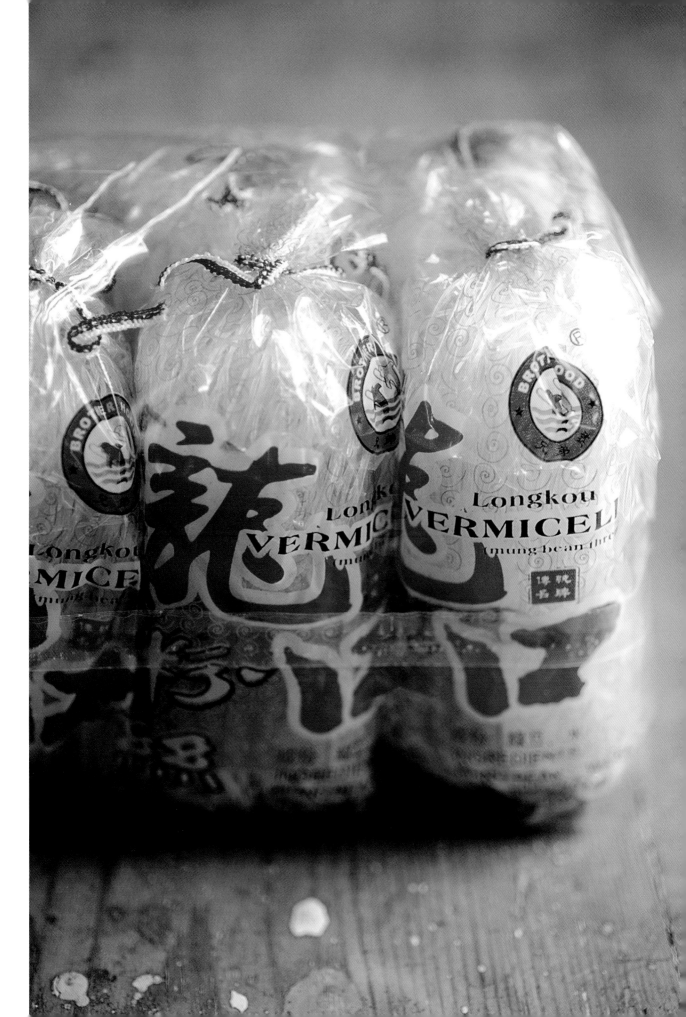

# Hot yogurt and fava bean soup

I came up with this soup when asked to contribute a seasonal recipe to the Royal Horticultural Society's flower show at Hampton Court Palace. It involves a bit of work but the result is, quite fittingly, majestic.

Serves 4

6 tbsp good-quality olive oil

1 medium onion, quartered

4 celery stalks, quartered

1 large carrot, peeled and cut into 1-inch chunks

5 thyme sprigs

2 bay leaves

½ cup flat-leaf parsley

1½ quarts water

3¼ cups shelled fava beans (fresh or frozen)

⅓ cup long-grain rice

salt and white pepper

2 cups Greek yogurt

2 garlic cloves, crushed

1 egg

3 tbsp roughly chopped dill

3 tbsp roughly chopped chervil

grated zest and juice of 1 lemon (optional)

Pour 2 tablespoons of the olive oil into a large pot. Heat up the oil and add the onion, celery and carrot. Sauté on medium heat for about 5 minutes; you want to soften up the vegetables without browning them. Next, add the thyme, bay leaves and parsley and cover with the water. Bring to the boil, then reduce the heat, cover and simmer gently for 30 minutes.

While the stock is cooking, get on with the arduous bit – preparing the fava beans. Bring a saucepan of water to the boil. Throw in the beans and simmer for just 1 minute. Drain, then refresh the beans under running cold water to stop the cooking. Next, remove the skins by gently pressing with your fingers against the sides of each bean, causing the soft bean to pop out; discard the skins.

When the stock is ready, pass it through a sieve into a medium saucepan; discard the vegetables and flavorings in the sieve. Add the rice to the stock. Bring to the boil, then simmer, covered, for 20 minutes. Now add half the skinned fava beans and some salt and pepper and use an immersion blender (or a regular blender) to blitz the soup until it is completely smooth.

Whisk together the yogurt, garlic and egg in a large heatproof bowl. Add a ladleful of the hot soup and whisk together. Continue gradually adding the soup until you've mixed in at least half of it. (It is important to do this slowly, otherwise the yogurt might split due to the difference in temperatures.)

Pour the tempered yogurt into the pan containing the rest of the soup. Place it on medium heat and warm up the soup while stirring constantly. Make sure the soup doesn't boil! Taste and add more salt and pepper, if you like.

Ladle the soup into four shallow bowls and drop in the remaining fava beans. Garnish generously with dill, chervil and lemon zest, and drizzle with the remaining 4 tablespoons olive oil (this is important), plus some lemon juice, if you like.

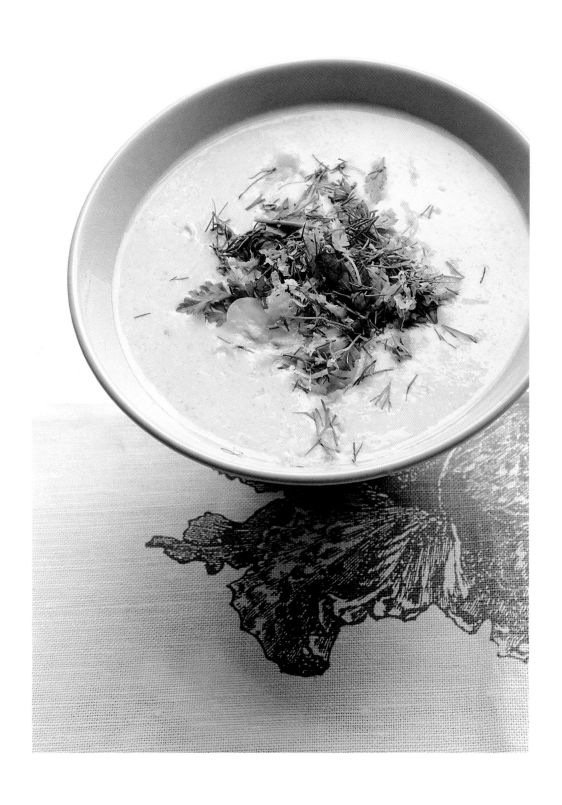

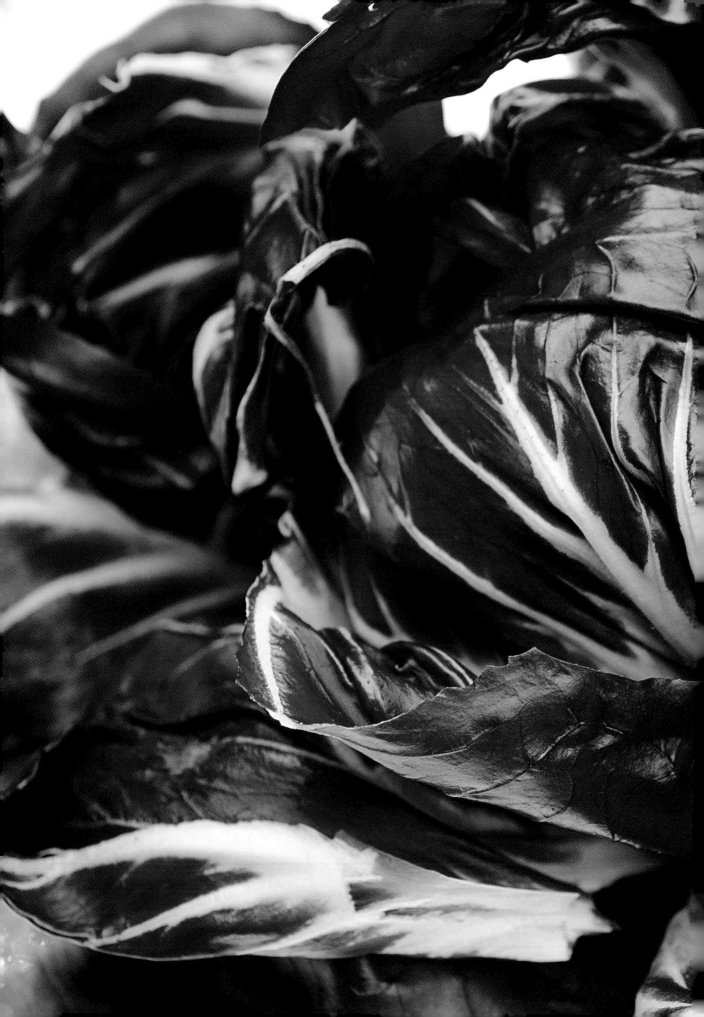

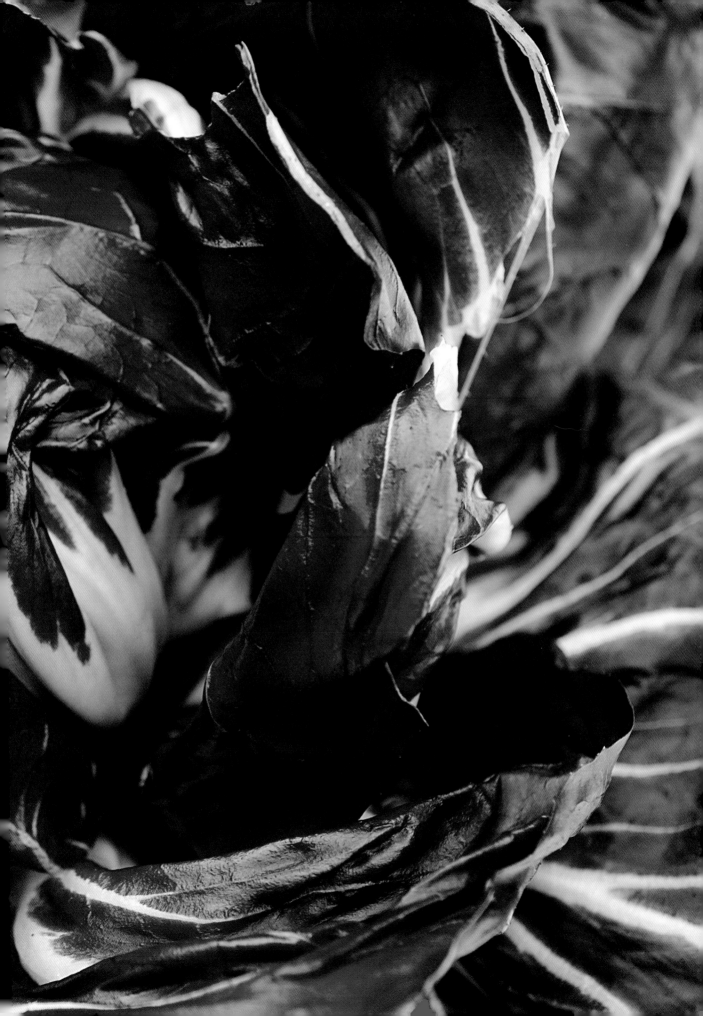

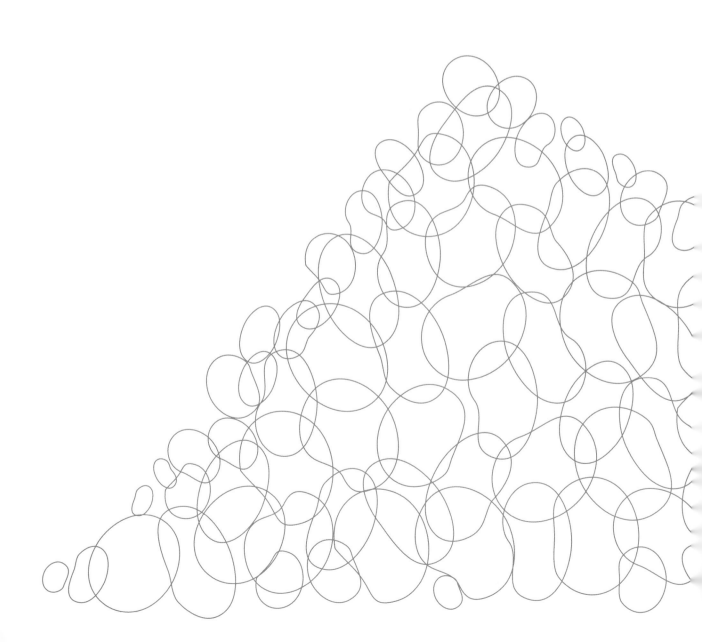

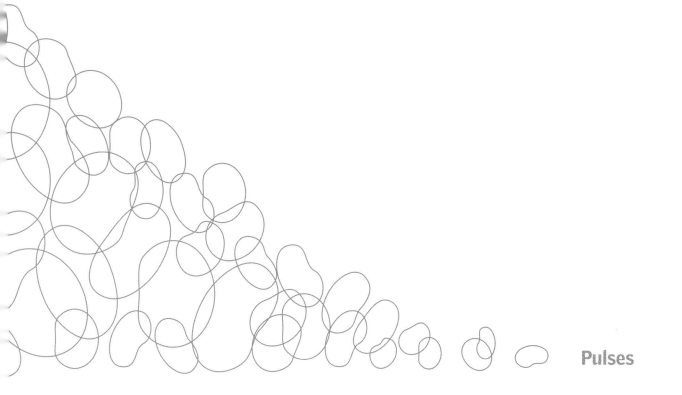

Pulses

# Puy lentil galettes

These may seem a bit outdated, reminiscent of the old vol-au-vents, but all good things eventually make a comeback and I am sure this modernized version will score you many points on the imaginative-host scale. The lentils are also delicious on their own, without the puff base.

You can skip the toasting and grinding of the seeds, if you prefer, and use ready-ground spices instead; just halve the quantity.

Serves 4
1 cup Puy lentils
2 bay leaves
2 tsp cumin seeds
2 tsp coriander seeds
5 tbsp olive oil, plus extra to finish
1 medium onion, roughly chopped
2 garlic cloves, crushed
1¼ cups Greek yogurt
2 cups baby spinach leaves
3 tbsp chopped cilantro
3 tbsp chopped mint
juice of 1 lemon
salt and black pepper
14 oz best-quality puff pastry
1 egg, beaten

Cook the lentils in a quart of boiling water with the bay leaves for 20 to 30 minutes, or until thoroughly cooked. Drain in a sieve and set aside.

In a small frying pan over medium heat, dry-roast the cumin and coriander seeds for 2 minutes, or until the aromas are released. Grind them using a mortar and pestle.

Heat 1 tablespoon of the olive oil in a small pan and fry the onion gently for 6 to 8 minutes, or until golden and very soft. Add the ground spices and garlic and cook for 2 more minutes. Mix this with the lentils and set aside to cool down. Once cool, stir in the yogurt, spinach, herbs, lemon juice and remaining olive oil. Taste and add salt and pepper.

Roll out the puff pastry 1¼ inches thick and cut out four circles about 3 inches in diameter. Place on a baking sheet and refrigerate for 30 minutes. Preheat the oven to 400°F.

Brush the pastry with the beaten egg and bake for 10 to 15 minutes, or until golden on top and underneath. Allow to cool slightly.

To serve, place the pastry discs in the middle of four serving plates. Pile up the lentils high on top so you can just see the edge of the pastry. Finish with a drizzle of olive oil.

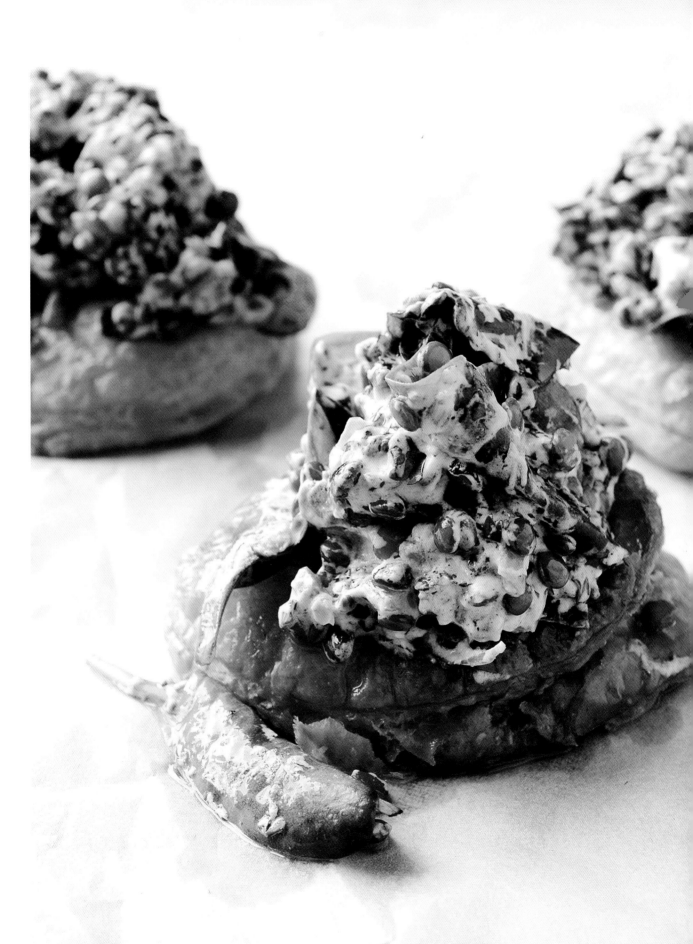

# Hummus with ful

When I am in Israel I often go to Abu Hassan in Jaffa, a tiny eatery where there is an endless line of Arabs and Jews standing at the door around lunchtime. It is one of those unique places I love so much, specializing in one thing and doing it to absolute perfection. Abu Hassan makes one of the best hummus in the world. Served warm with *ful*, which is a hearty paste of dried fava beans, this is a popular breakfast or lunch dish among Lebanese, Palestinians, Syrians and Israelis. Served with warm pita, raw onion and hard-boiled egg, it isn't the lightest affair, but it's completely delicious. For a simpler experience, make only the hummus (pictured on page 212) and serve it warm or chilled (it can be kept in the fridge for up to 2 days).

Serves 6
2½ cups dried chickpeas
1½ tbsp baking soda
1¼ cups tahini paste
3 tbsp lemon juice
6 garlic cloves, crushed
salt

Ful
1½ cups dried fava beans
⅓ cup olive oil
⅓ cup lemon juice
1 tbsp ground cumin
4 garlic cloves, crushed
1 tsp salt

⅓ cup olive oil
⅓ cup lemon juice
1 tsp sweet paprika
6 tbsp roughly chopped parsley
     (optional)
3 eggs, hard-boiled and quartered
1 medium onion, cut into 6 wedges
     (optional)

Soak the chickpeas and fava beans overnight. Place them in two separate bowls and cover with double their volume of cold water. Add 1 tablespoon baking soda to the chickpeas. Set both aside. The next day, drain and rinse both.

Place the soaked chickpeas and remaining baking soda in a medium saucepan and cover with double their volume of cold water. Bring to the boil, then simmer very gently for 2 to 3 hours, or until totally soft and easy to mush. Add more water during cooking if necessary, to keep them immersed. Drain them, retaining the cooking liquid.

Transfer the warm chickpeas to a food processor, reserving a few to garnish at the end, and add the tahini, lemon juice, garlic and 1 teaspoon salt. Blitz for a minute or two until totally smooth. Add some of the cooking liquid and blitz again. You want the mixture to be very soft, almost runny, but just holding its shape. Taste and add more salt if you like. Keep warm.

To make the ful. Place the fava beans in a medium saucepan and cover with double their volume of water. Simmer gently for about 3 hours (they may take longer), adding more water if necessary. By the end of the cooking time, hardly any liquid should be left in the pan (drain it out if needed) and the beans should have begun to disintegrate, or will do so easily when crushed with a fork. Remove from the heat and add the olive oil, lemon juice, cumin, garlic and salt. Taste and adjust the seasoning.

To serve, spread the warm hummus in small individual plates. Spoon the ful in the center and drizzle the olive oil and lemon juice on top and around. Sprinkle with paprika, garnish with the reserved chickpeas, plenty of parsley, if using, and serve egg and onion on the side.

# Chickpea sauté with Greek yogurt

This is a quick and simple dish (pictured on page 213) that is nice both warm and at room temperature. When chard isn't in season try a combination of spinach and arugula (you won't need to blanch them) and sprinkle with sumac or ground Persian lime (see page 245).

Serves 4
¾ lb (8 cups) Swiss chard
⅓ cup olive oil, plus extra to finish
4 medium carrots, peeled and cut into
⅜-inch dice
1 tsp caraway seeds
1½ cups freshly cooked chickpeas
(canned are fine too)
1 garlic clove, crushed
1 tbsp chopped mint
1 tbsp chopped cilantro
1 tbsp lemon juice
salt and black pepper
½ cup Greek yogurt
1 tbsp olive oil

Separate the chard stalks from the leaves. Blanch the stalks in plenty of boiling salted water for 3 minutes. Add the leaves and continue cooking for 2 minutes, then drain everything. Refresh under cold running water and squeeze dry, then chop roughly.

Heat up the olive oil in a large, heavy saucepan. Add the carrots and caraway seeds and sauté for 5 minutes on medium heat. Add the chard and chickpeas and continue cooking for 6 minutes. Now add the garlic, herbs, lemon juice and some salt and pepper. Remove from the heat and cool down a little. Taste and adjust the seasoning.

To serve, mix together the yogurt, olive oil and some salt and pepper. Pile the vegetables on serving dishes and spoon the yogurt on top. Sprinkle with freshly ground pepper and drizzle over more olive oil.

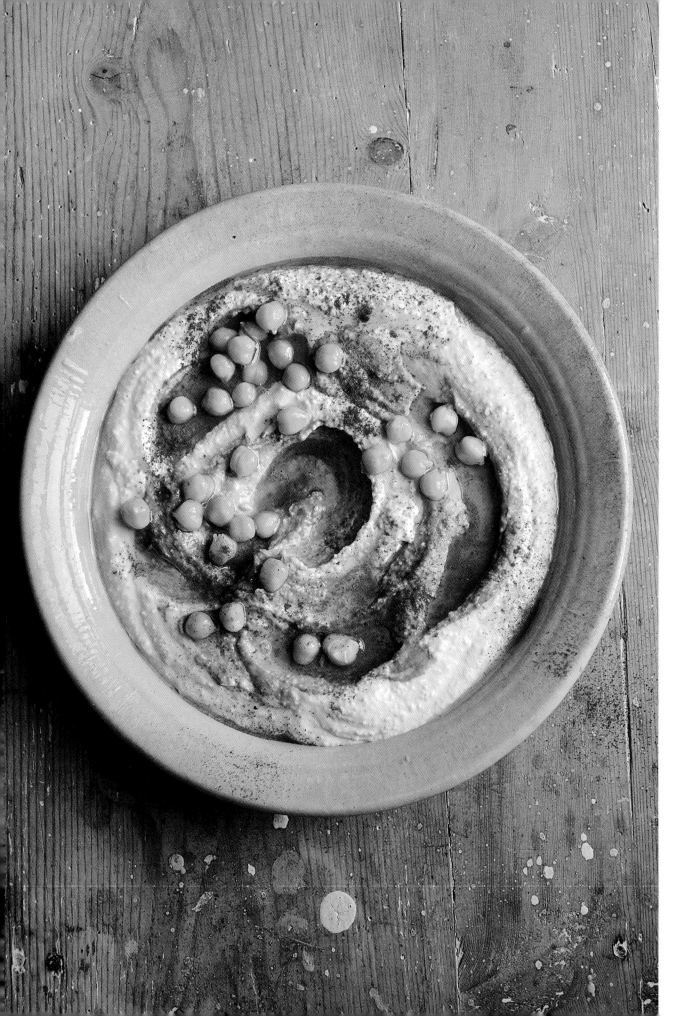

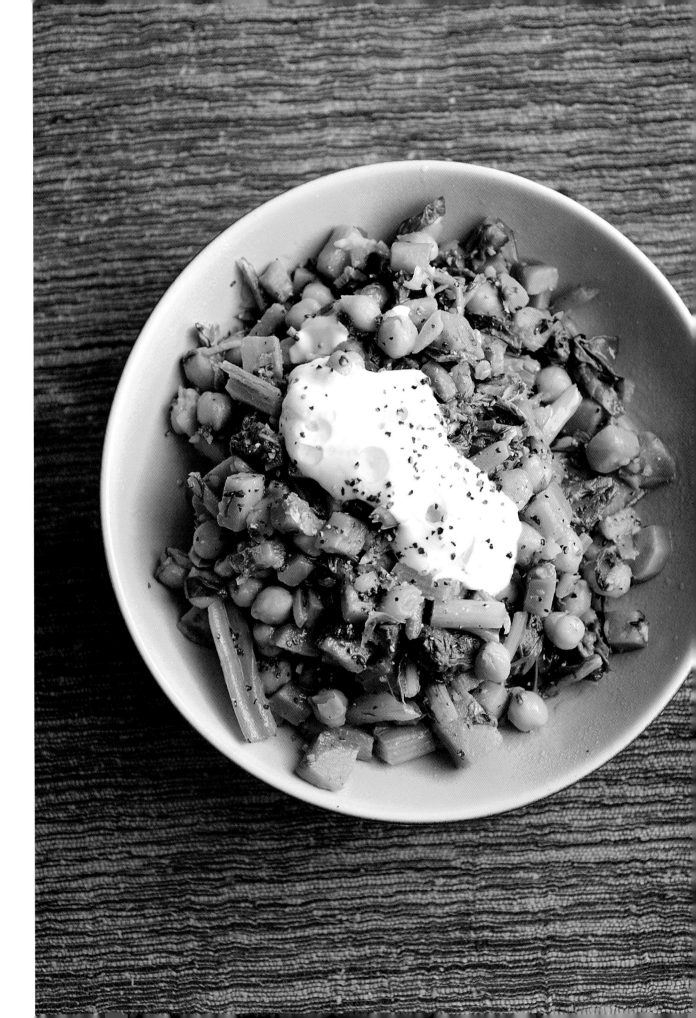

# Fried lima beans with feta, sorrel and sumac

I knew something was achieved when I recently spotted sumac in the spice section of my local supermarket. Who had even heard of sumac, or za'atar, a couple of years ago? Although I can't take full credit for it, this is a first step toward introducing a new exciting spice to the home cook and my answer to skeptics who often ask me why I use all these exotic ingredients that are impossible to find. Just in case you don't live near me, you can get both za'atar and sumac from Middle Eastern shops, or buy them online from penzeys.com. If you can't find sorrel, use spinach and double the amount of lemon juice.

Serves 4

1 lb dried lima beans
2 tbsp baking soda
1½ tbsp butter
4 tbsp olive oil, plus extra to finish
8 green onions, sliced lengthways into
    long strips
1 garlic clove, crushed
2 fresh red chiles, thinly sliced (optional)
5 cups sorrel, cut into ¾-inch strips,
    plus extra very thinly sliced to finish
½ tsp salt
1½ tbsp lemon juice
5 oz feta, crumbled
2 tsp sumac
handful of chopped soft herbs such as
    dill or chervil

Place the lima beans in a large bowl and add twice their volume of cold water and the baking soda. Leave to soak overnight.

The following day, drain the beans, place in a large pan and cover with plenty of fresh water. Bring to the boil and boil for at least 30 minutes, or until soft to the bite but not disintegrating. They could take over an hour to cook, depending on size and freshness. Add more water during cooking if necessary. When ready, drain the beans.

Next, you want to lightly fry them. You may need to do this in three or four batches, depending on the size of your pan. Take some of the butter and oil and heat up well. Add enough beans to cover the bottom of the pan and fry on medium–high heat for 1 to 2 minutes on each side, or until the skin is golden brown and blistered. Remove to a large bowl and continue with another batch of butter, oil and beans.

When cooking the final batch, as soon as the beans are almost done, add the green onions, garlic, chiles, if using, and sorrel and sauté for about a minute. Then add the rest of the beans to the pan, remove from the heat and season with the salt. Allow the beans to cool down completely or until just warmish.

Taste the beans for seasoning, drizzle some lemon juice on top, then scatter with feta, a sprinkling of sumac, chopped herbs and some thinly sliced sorrel. Finish with a drizzle of olive oil.

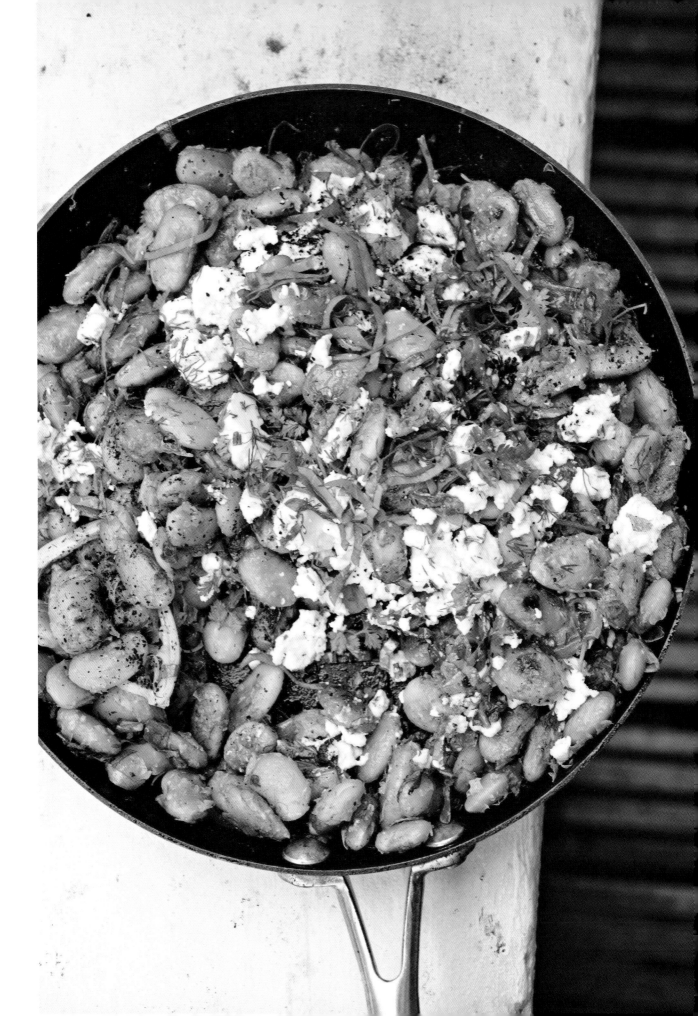

# Celeriac and lentils with hazelnut and mint

Celeriac is probably my favorite root. It is delicate, yet very nutty, and has an elegant oily smoothness. Like all good vegetables, it is marvelous simply with a bit of olive oil. Here it works with the lentils and nuts to create a hearty autumn main course. Serve it warm, with a radish, cucumber and dill salad dressed with sour cream and olive oil. Or allow it to cool down, then take it to work for lunch or on a picnic.

Serves 4

⅓ cup whole hazelnuts (skin on)
1 cup Puy lentils
3 cups water
2 bay leaves
4 thyme sprigs
1 small celeriac (1½ lbs), peeled and cut
    into ⅜-inch chips
4 tbsp olive oil
3 tbsp hazelnut oil
3 tbsp good-quality red wine vinegar
salt and black pepper
4 tbsp chopped mint

Preheat the oven to 275°F. Scatter the hazelnuts on a small baking sheet and roast in the oven for 15 minutes. Let them cool down, then chop roughly.

Combine the lentils, water, bay leaves and thyme in a small saucepan. Bring to the boil, then simmer for 15 to 20 minutes, or until al dente. Drain in a sieve.

Meanwhile, in a separate saucepan, cook the celeriac in plenty of boiling salted water for 8 to 12 minutes, or until just tender. Drain.

In a large bowl mix the hot lentils (if they have cooled down they won't soak up all the flavors) with the olive oil, 2 tablespoons of the hazelnut oil, the vinegar, plenty of salt and some black pepper. Add the celeriac and stir well. Taste and adjust the seasoning.

To serve right away, stir in half the mint and half the hazelnuts. Pile onto a serving dish or in a bowl and drizzle the remaining hazelnut oil on top. Garnish with the rest of the mint and hazelnuts.

To serve cold, wait for the lentils and celeriac to cool down before finally adjusting the seasoning and possibly adding some more vinegar, if you like. Add hazelnut oil, mint and nuts in the same way as when serving hot.

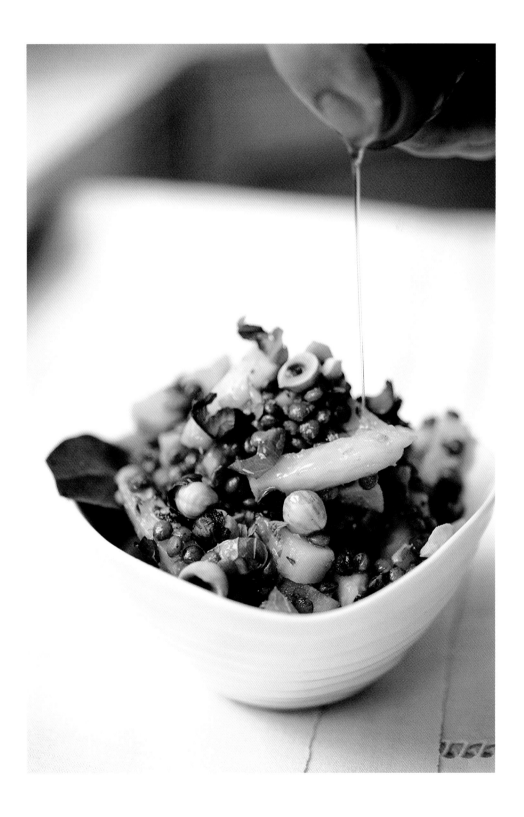

# Chickpea, tomato and bread soup

Here's a take on the Tuscan *ribollita*. Somewhere between a soup and a vegetable stew, it is a warming and filling meal in a bowl after which you don't need much – maybe just a little pillow to rest your head on. You can reduce or increase the amount of liquid to achieve your perfect consistency.

Serves 4–6

1 large onion, sliced

1 medium fennel bulb, sliced

about ½ cup olive oil

1 large carrot, peeled, cut lengthways in
    half and sliced

3 celery stalks, sliced

1 tbsp tomato paste

1 cup white wine

one 14-oz can Italian plum tomatoes

1 tbsp chopped oregano

2 tbsp chopped parsley

1 tbsp thyme leaves

2 bay leaves

2 tsp sugar

4½ cups vegetable stock

salt and black pepper

2 large slices stale sourdough bread
    (crust removed)

2½ cups freshly cooked chickpeas
    (canned are fine too)

4 tbsp basil pesto (bought or freshly
    made; see Royal Potato Salad,
    page 20)

handful of shredded basil leaves to serve
    (optional)

Preheat the oven to 350°F. Place the onion and fennel in a large saucepan, add 3 tablespoons of the oil and sauté on medium heat for about 4 minutes. Add the carrot and celery and continue cooking for 4 minutes, just to soften the vegetables, stirring occasionally. Stir in the tomato paste and stir as you cook for 1 minute. Add the wine and let it bubble away for a minute or two.

Next, add the canned tomatoes with their juices, the herbs, sugar, vegetable stock and some salt and pepper. Bring to the boil, then cover and leave to simmer gently for about 30 minutes.

While you wait, break the bread into rough chunks with your hands. Toss with 2 tablespoons oil and some salt and scatter in a roasting pan. Bake for about 10 minutes, or until thoroughly dry. Remove from the oven and set aside.

About 10 minutes before you want to serve the soup, place the chickpeas in a bowl and crush them a little with a potato masher or the end of a rolling pin; you want some to be left whole. Add them to the soup and leave to simmer for a further 5 minutes. Next add the toasted bread, stir well and cook for another 5 minutes. Taste the soup and add salt and pepper liberally.

Ladle the hot soup into bowls. Spoon some pesto in the center, drizzle with plenty of olive oil and finish with a generous amount of freshly shredded basil, if you like.

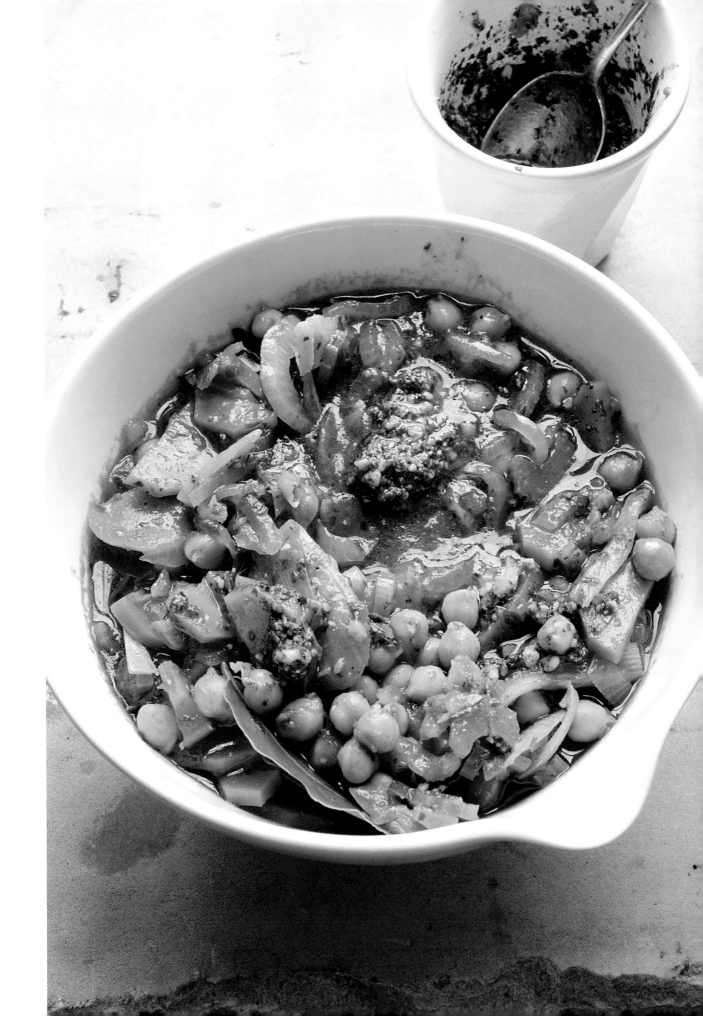

# Green lentils, asparagus and watercress

When this recipe was first published I used young pecorino cheese in it so as not to outdo the asparagus. I have since realized that fresh asparagus actually withstands quite a lot and can impart its flavor over pretty gutsy dishes. A flavorful sheep's cheese is ideal with the earthy lentils.

Serves 4 generously
1 cup green lentils
4 cups watercress (thick stalks removed)
⅔ cup parsley
⅔ cup light olive oil
1 tbsp red wine vinegar
1 garlic clove, peeled
salt and black pepper
1 large bunch thin asparagus spears
3½ oz semi-mature pecorino (or one of the more full-bodied varieties of Manchego), broken into chunks
walnut oil to finish (optional)
4 lemon wedges

Wash the lentils in cold water, then place in a saucepan with plenty of fresh water and bring to the boil. Simmer for 15 minutes, or until the lentils are just cooked but haven't started to disintegrate.

While the lentils are cooking, put half the watercress, the parsley, olive oil, vinegar, garlic and some salt and pepper into a food processor. Blitz until smooth. Pour into a bowl.

As soon as the lentils are cooked drain them well and mix them, while still hot, with the watercress dressing. Taste and adjust the seasoning; you will probably need more salt.

Cook the asparagus in simmering salted water for 2 to 3 minutes; drain. Cut the spears into roughly 2½-inch-long segments.

You can serve the salad warm or at room temperature. Toss together the lentils, asparagus and most of the remaining watercress. Add pieces of cheese as you plate the salad. Drizzle with walnut oil, if using, and garnish with the reserved watercress. Serve with wedges of lemon.

# Spiced red lentils with cucumber yogurt

My friend and colleague, Helen Goh, is a bit of food encyclopedia. I am always astounded by how much she knows and how effortlessly she accesses her knowledge. After suggesting that I try this dish, which she hadn't cooked for years, Helen went on to rapidly recite the long list of ingredients and quantities as if she were reading from her notes. She didn't miss a single item!

Serves 2–4

1 cup split red lentils
1½ cups water
1 bunch cilantro (3½ cups), plus extra
    leaves to garnish
1 small onion, peeled
2½ inches peeled fresh ginger
3 garlic cloves, peeled
1 mild fresh green chile
1½ tsp black mustard seeds
4 tbsp sunflower oil
1½ tsp ground coriander
1 tsp ground cumin
½ tsp ground turmeric
¼ tsp sweet paprika
10 curry leaves
1¾ cups peeled chopped tomatoes
    (fresh or canned)
2 tsp sugar
¼ tsp fenugreek (optional)
pinch of asafetida (optional)
salt
¾ cup Greek yogurt
¾ cup finely diced cucumber
1½ tbsp olive oil
⅓ cup unsalted butter
1½ tbsp lime juice

Wash the lentils under plenty of running cold water, then soak in the 1½ cups of water for 30 minutes.

Cut the cilantro bunch somewhere around its center to get a leafy top half and a stalk and root half. Chop up the leaves roughly; set aside. Place the stalk ends in a food processor bowl and add the onion, ginger, garlic and chile – all roughly broken. Pulse a few times to chop up everything without turning them into a paste.

Put the mustard seeds in a heavy pot and set on medium heat. When they begin to pop, add the chopped onion mix and the sunflower oil. Reduce heat to low and cook, stirring, for about 10 minutes. Add the ground coriander, cumin, turmeric, paprika and curry leaves, and continue cooking and stirring for 5 minutes.

Next, add the lentils and their soaking water, the tomatoes, sugar, fenugreek, and asafetida, if using, and some salt. Cover and simmer for about 30 minutes, or until the lentils are fully cooked.

Meanwhile, whisk together the yogurt, cucumber, olive oil and some salt.

Stir the butter, lime juice and chopped cilantro leaves into the lentils; taste and season generously with salt. Divide among bowls, spoon the yogurt on top and garnish with cilantro leaves.

# Castelluccio lentils with tomatoes and Gorgonzola

Castelluccio lentils from Umbria are tiny brownish jewels with a delicate flavor and a wonderfully tender texture. Like Puy lentils, they don't disintegrate in the cooking, which makes them ideal for salads. You can get them from Italian or gourmet markets, or use Puy instead. This substantial dish, which is best eaten at room temperature, can be served on its own or with steamed seasonal greens such as broccolini or baby fennel.

Serves 4

**Oven-dried tomatoes**

5 plum tomatoes

8 thyme sprigs

1 tbsp olive oil

2 tbsp balsamic vinegar

salt

1 small red onion, very thinly sliced

1 tbsp good-quality red wine vinegar

1 tsp Maldon sea salt

1⅓ cups Castelluccio lentils

3 tbsp olive oil

1 garlic clove, crushed

black pepper

3 tbsp chopped chervil or parsley

3 tbsp chopped chives

4 tbsp chopped dill

3 oz mild Gorgonzola, crumbled

To make the oven-dried tomatoes. Preheat the oven to 275°F. Quarter the tomatoes vertically and place skin-side down on a baking sheet lined with parchment paper. Arrange the thyme sprigs on top of them. Drizzle over the olive oil and balsamic vinegar and sprinkle with some salt. Roast for 1½ hours, or until semi-dried. Discard the thyme and allow to cool down slightly.

Meanwhile, place the red onion in a medium bowl, pour over the vinegar and sprinkle with the sea salt. Stir, then leave for a few minutes so the onion softens a bit.

Place the lentils in a pan of boiling water (the water should come 1¼ inches above the lentils) and cook for 20 to 30 minutes, or until tender. Drain well in a sieve and, while still warm, add to the sliced onion. Also add the olive oil, garlic and some black pepper. Stir to mix and leave aside to cool down. Once cool, add the herbs and gently mix together. Taste and adjust the seasoning.

To serve, pile up the lentils on a large plate or bowl, integrating the Gorgonzola and tomatoes as you build up the pile. Drizzle the tomato cooking juices on top and serve.

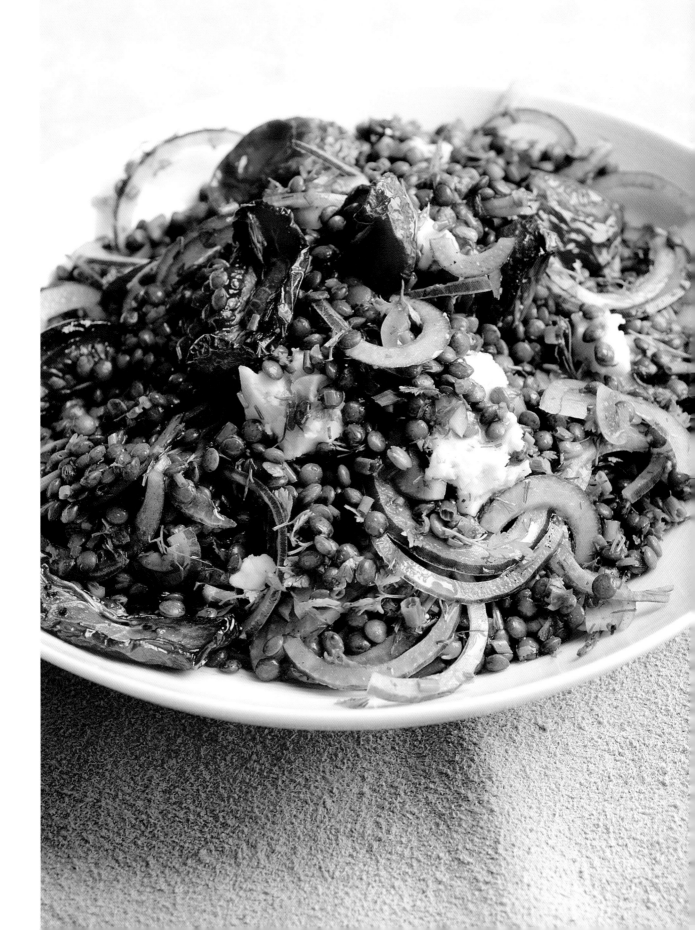

# Socca

On a visit to southern France my partner, Karl, and I were taken to Grain de Sel, a minute restaurant in the village of Cogolin, run by an inspiring couple, Anne and Philippe Audibert. Among other brilliant dishes made from local produce that Philippe buys daily in the local market, I was served a variation on the renowned pissaladière. Instead of the normal dough base, Philippe used socca batter, a speciality of Nice made from chickpea flour, water and olive oil. He was generous enough to give me the recipe.

Serves 4
2 cups cherry tomatoes, halved
5½ tbsp olive oil, plus more for drizzling
1¾ lbs white onions, cut into thin rings
2 tbsp thyme leaves
salt and black pepper
½ tsp white wine vinegar
1¾ cups chickpea flour
2 cups water
2 egg whites
crème fraîche to serve

Preheat the oven to 275°F. Spread the tomatoes cut-side up on a small baking pan and sprinkle them with some salt and pepper and a drizzle of oil. Roast for 25 minutes, or until semi-cooked. They are not supposed to dry out completely.

Meanwhile, heat up 4 tablespoons olive oil in a large frying pan. Add the onions, thyme and some salt and pepper and cook on high heat, stirring, for about a minute. Reduce the heat to low and continue cooking for 20 minutes, stirring occasionally. You want the onions completely soft, sweet and golden brown, but not very dark. At the end, stir in the vinegar, then taste and adjust the seasoning.

When you take the tomatoes out of the oven, increase the temperature to 325°F.

Put the chickpea flour, water, 1½ tablespoons olive oil, ¾ teaspoon salt and some pepper in a bowl. Mix well with a hand whisk until the batter is totally homogenous. In a separate bowl whisk the egg whites to soft peaks and gently fold into the batter.

Line two baking sheets with parchment paper and brush the paper with a little bit of oil; set on the side. Then take a small nonstick frying pan, roughly 6 inches diameter at its base, and brush it with the smallest amount of olive oil. Put on high heat for a couple of minutes, then reduce heat to medium–high and pour in one-quarter of the socca batter. It should be about scant ¼ inch thick. After about 2 minutes air bubbles will appear on the surface and the pancake will have set on its base. Use an offset spatula to release its edges from the pan, then carefully lift and turn it over. Cook for another minute. Transfer to the lined baking sheet. Repeat with the rest of the batter. When all the pancakes have been made, place in the oven for 5 minutes.

To serve, spread the onion over the pancakes; they should be totally covered. Arrange tomato halves on top. Place in the oven to warm up for about 4 minutes. Serve warm, with crème fraîche on the side.

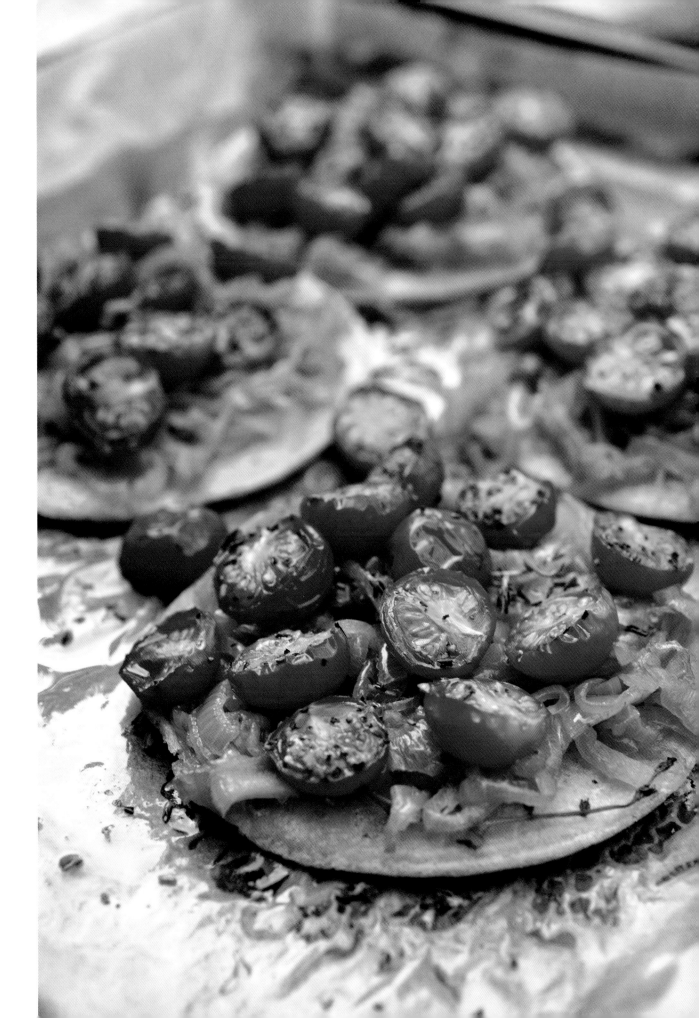

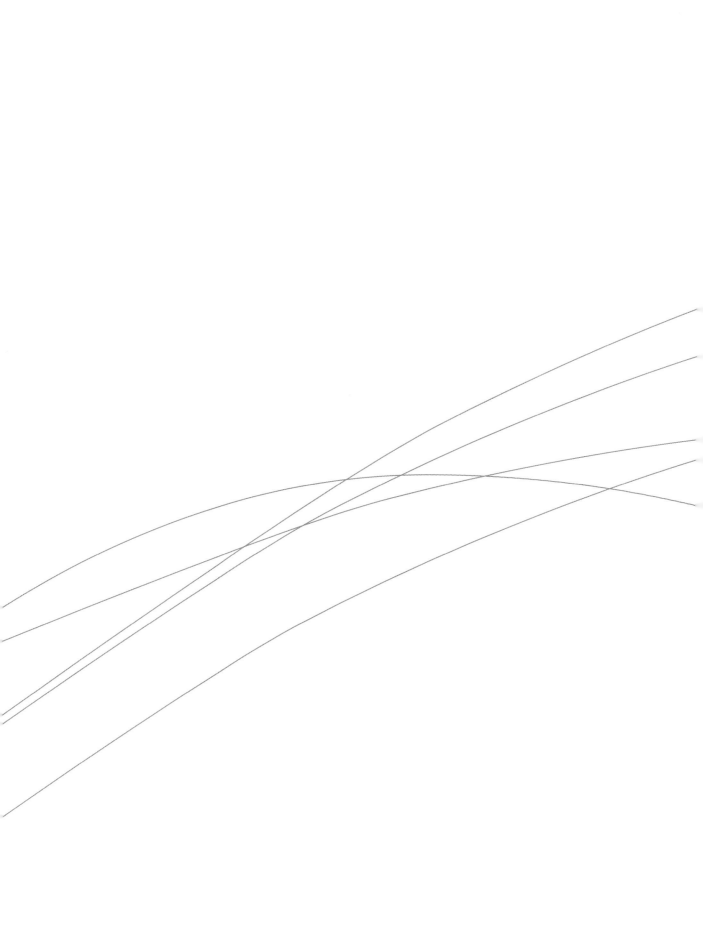

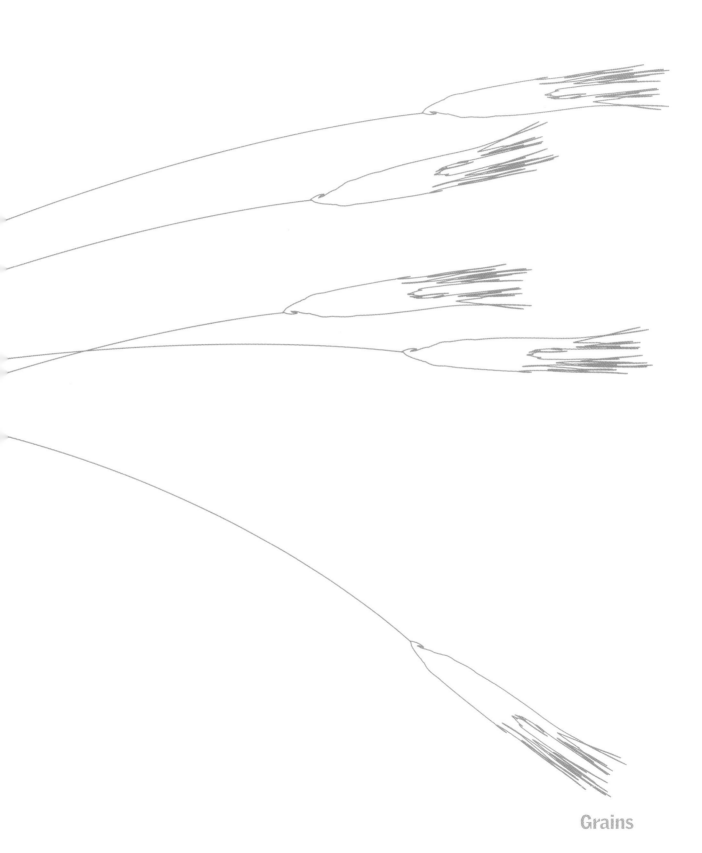

Grains

# Avocado, quinoa and fava bean salad

A simple salad for a spring brunch. Serve it with good bread and that's it.

Serves 6

1 cup quinoa

1 lb (3 cups) shelled fava beans (fresh or frozen)

2 medium lemons

2 small ripe avocados

2 garlic cloves, crushed

2 bunches breakfast radishes, halved lengthways

1 cup purple radish cress (or small purple basil leaves)

1 tbsp ground cumin

⅓ cup olive oil

¼ tsp chile flakes

salt and black pepper

Place the quinoa in a saucepan with plenty of water, bring to the boil and simmer for 9 minutes. Drain in a fine sieve, rinse under cold water and leave to dry.

Throw the fava beans into a pan of boiling water, bring back to the boil and immediately drain in a colander. Refresh with cold water and leave to dry. Then gently press each bean with your fingers to remove the skins; discard these.

Take the lemons and use a small sharp knife to slice off the top and base. Stand each one on a chopping board and cut down the sides, following the natural curve, to remove the skin and white pith. Over a large mixing bowl, cut in between the membranes to release the individual segments into the bowl. Squeeze the juice from the membrane into the bowl with the segments.

Peel and stone the avocados. Slice thinly, then add to the bowl and toss to cover in the lemon juice. Once the quinoa is dry, transfer it to the bowl. Add the fava beans, garlic, radishes, half the radish cress, the cumin, olive oil, chile flakes and some salt and pepper. Toss very gently, without breaking the avocado. Taste and add more salt and pepper, if you wish. Plate and garnish with the remaining cress.

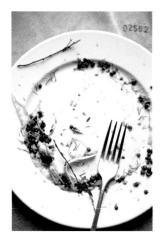

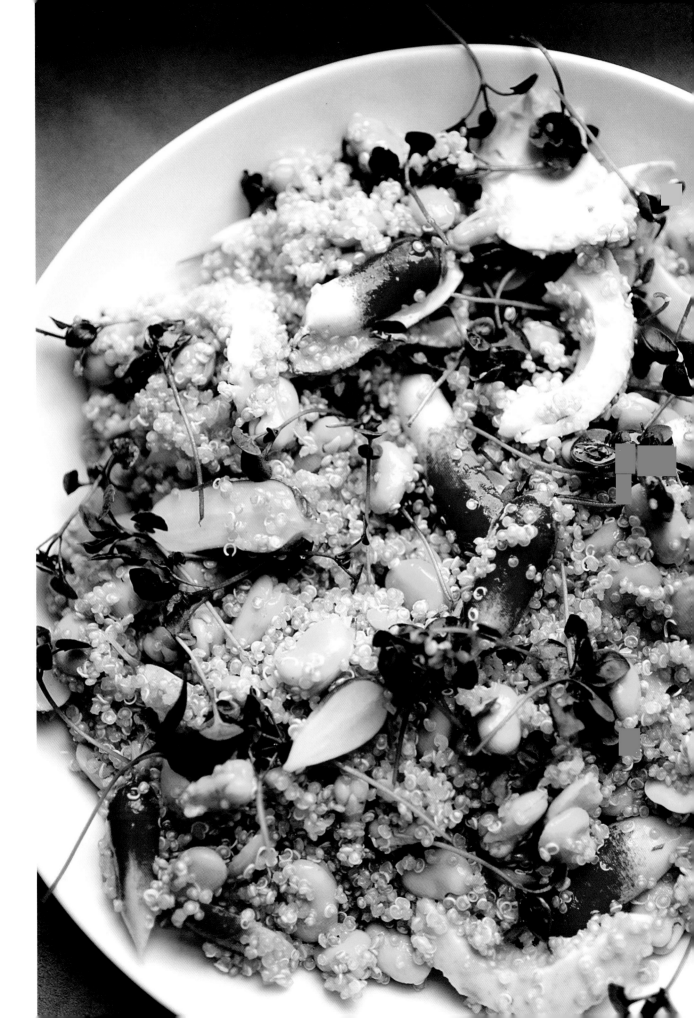

# Coconut rice with sambal and okra

Breakfast is the one meal in the day when cultural boundaries aren't easily crossed – even the most experimental and daring of eaters revert to what they know and like, which is their mom's cooking. My friend Helen Goh, who was brought up in Malaysia, finds it excruciatingly difficult to have anything in the morning but the national breakfast grub, nasi lemak. Nothing else turns her on. My dish (pictured on page 232) is inspired by nasi lemak. I dare you to serve it for breakfast! And be warned: it is very hot.

Crisp-fried shallots are available from Asian grocers. You can also make them yourself, or substitute dried onion flakes.

Serves 4
**Sambal**
5 fresh red chiles (1 oz in total), seeded
5 dried red chiles (⅛ oz in total), seeded
20 baby shallots (4 oz in total), peeled
1 garlic clove, peeled
½ tsp salt
½ cup vegetable oil
2 tbsp water
1 tbsp thick tamarind water (seedless tamarind pulp whisked with a little water, then strained)
1 tbsp sugar

**Rice**
1⅔ cups basmati rice
½ tsp salt
¾ cup coconut milk
1½ cups water
6 kaffir lime leaves (optional)
6 thin slices of fresh ginger

1¼ lbs (6 cups) okra, trimmed (see page 179)
2 tbsp crisp-fried shallots
large handful of roughly chopped cilantro
2 limes, halved

To make the sambal. Place the fresh and dried chiles, shallots, garlic and salt in a food processor and add 2 tablespoons of the oil and the water. Blitz for about a minute, or until you get a fine paste (this can also be made using a mortar and pestle but without the liquids; add these once you have a paste).

Set a wok or a large heavy frying pan on high heat. Once hot, add the remaining oil and heat up well. Now add the chile paste and stir. Reduce the heat at once to avoid burning and cook on a low simmer, stirring frequently, for 5 to 10 minutes, or until you get a beautiful dark-red oily paste. Off the heat, stir in the tamarind water and sugar. Set aside.

To make the rice. Wash the rice well under plenty of cold running water. Drain well and put into a medium saucepan. Heat the rice up a little, then add the salt, coconut milk, water, lime leaves and ginger. Stir and bring to the boil. Reduce the heat to a minimum, cover and leave to simmer for 12 minutes. Remove from the heat and leave, covered, for 10 minutes. Before serving, fluff up the rice with a fork.

While the rice is cooking bring a medium pan of water to the boil. Throw the okra into the boiling water and cook for 2 to 3 minutes only, so it remains firm. Drain, rinse under cold running water and leave to dry.

When you are ready to serve, reheat the sambal in its pan. Add the okra and stir just to warm it up (don't cook it any more). Spoon some rice into each serving bowl or plate. Top with okra and sambal, and sprinkle with fried shallots and chopped cilantro. Place a lime half on the side of each bowl and encourage everybody to squeeze its juice liberally on top.

# Lemon and eggplant risotto

The crucial component in this dish is the stock, which will make or break it. You can quickly make one by covering some aromatic vegetables and herbs (carrot, celery, onion, bay leaf, parsley, garlic, lemongrass, fennel, thyme, etc.) with water and simmering for half an hour. Look at the Parsnip Dumplings in Broth on page 28 for a lengthier version. Unlike some other risotti, this one (pictured on page 233) feels light as a feather – or almost.

Serves 4
2 medium eggplants
½ cup plus 1 tbsp olive oil
coarse sea salt
1 medium onion, finely chopped
2 garlic cloves, crushed
7 oz good-quality risotto rice
½ cup white wine
3¼ cups hot vegetable stock
grated zest of 1 lemon
2 tbsp lemon juice
1½ tbsp butter
½ cup grated Parmesan (about 2 oz)
    (or another mature hard cheese)
black pepper
½ cup shredded basil leaves

Start by burning one of the eggplants (see page 116). Once ready, remove from the heat and make a long cut through the eggplant. Scoop out the soft flesh while avoiding the skin. Discard the skin. Chop the flesh roughly and set aside.

Cut the other eggplant into ½-inch dice. Heat up ⅓ cup of the olive oil in a frying pan and fry the eggplant dice in batches until golden and crisp. Transfer to a colander and sprinkle with salt. Leave to cool.

Put the onion and remaining oil in a heavy pan and fry slowly until soft and translucent. Add the garlic and cook for a further 3 minutes. Turn up the heat and add the rice, stirring to coat it in the oil. Fry for 2 to 3 minutes. Add the wine (it should hiss) and cook for 2 to 3 minutes, or until nearly evaporated. Turn the heat down to medium.

Now start adding the hot stock to the rice, a ladleful at a time, waiting until each addition has been fully absorbed before adding the next and stirring all the time. When all the stock has been added, remove the pan from the heat. Add half the lemon zest, the lemon juice, grilled eggplant, butter, most of the Parmesan and ¾ teaspoon salt. Stir well, then cover and set aside for 5 minutes. Taste and add more salt, if you like, plus some black pepper.

To serve, spoon the risotto into shallow bowls and sprinkle with the diced eggplant, the remaining Parmesan, the basil and the rest of the lemon zest.

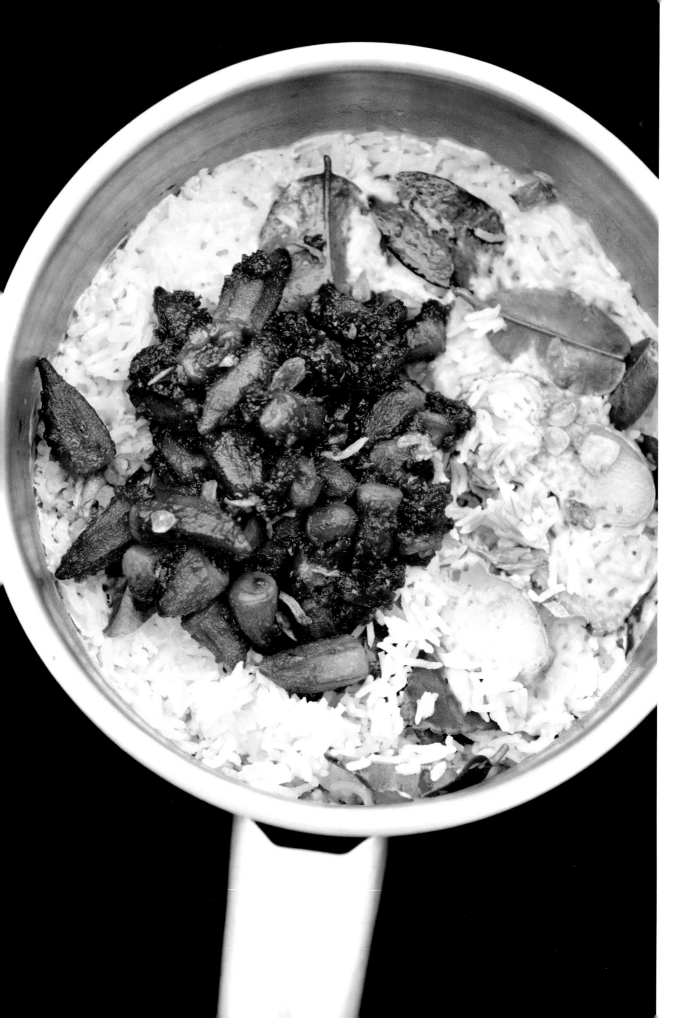

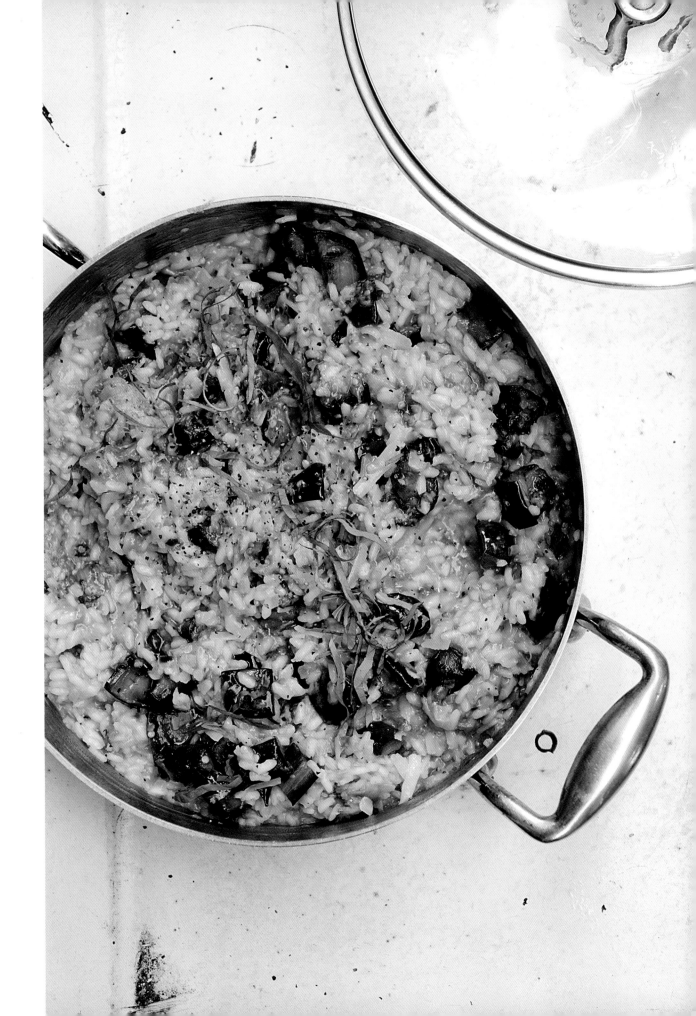

# Farro and roasted pepper salad

I first tried farro when my friend and ex-colleague, Nir Feller, cooked with it at Ottolenghi in Notting Hill. Initially I wasn't quite sold on it; it just tasted a bit too "healthy" for my liking. Since then, though, I have grown to appreciate farro's nutty aroma and its robust texture that goes so well with intense flavors.

Farro is the Italian name for an old wheat variety similar to, or possibly even the same as, emmer or spelt. It can be eaten by some people who are normally intolerant of wheat. It is sold in a few forms – whole, semi-pearled and pearled – and the one you use will determine the cooking time, which is anywhere from 15 minutes to an hour. When done it should be tender but retain a real bite. Get it in Italian or well-stocked supermarkets. Alternatively, use pearled spelt or pearl barley.

Serves 4 as a starter

**Dressing**
juice of 1 medium lemon
3 tbsp olive oil
1 tbsp honey
¼ tsp ground allspice
¼ tsp smoked paprika, plus extra to garnish
½ garlic clove, crushed
¼ tsp fine sea salt

¾ cup farro
2 red bell peppers
10 pitted black olives, quartered lengthways
1 tbsp chopped fresh oregano or picked thyme leaves
3 green onions, thinly sliced
4 oz feta, crumbled

To make the dressing. Whisk together all the ingredients in a bowl and set aside.

Bring a large pot of water to a boil. Add farro and simmer until just tender. Drain in a sieve, rinse under cold water and set aside.

Preheat a grill pan to high. Use a small, sharp knife to cut around the stem of each bell pepper and lift it out with the seeds attached. Put the peppers on the grill pan and grill, turning them every now and then, until they are totally black on the outside; this will take 30 minutes or more. When ready, remove the pan from the heat and cover it with foil. Once the peppers are cool enough to handle, remove and discard the skin. Tear them by hand into roughly ⅜-inch-wide slices.

Place the cooked farro in a large mixing bowl and add the peppers, olives, oregano or thyme, green onions and most of the feta, reserving some to finish. Pour over the dressing and gently mix everything together. Taste and add more salt if you like.

To serve, pile up the salad on a plate or in a bowl and finish with the reserved feta and a sprinkle of paprika.

# Steamed rice with herbs (or, actually, herbs with rice)

This Iranian rice, called *sabzi polo*, is normally served with fish but works well with almost anything else and also on its own with just a condiment. Instead of the yogurt and cream condiment you can serve tzatziki or a sweetish tomato sauce (see Okra with Tomato, Lemon and Cilantro, page 179, with or without the okra).

The method I describe is very particular but it is essential you stick to it to get incredibly light and fluffy steamed rice. There are also heaps of herbs here, reversing the usual proportions of herbs to the rest, which gives the rice its distinct earthy aroma. Buy your herbs from a greengrocer or farmers' market, or you'll need dozens of the minuscule supermarket-size bunches. Although I always prefer manual chopping of herbs, you can save your muscles by using a food processor in this case.

Serves 4 as a side dish

1¼ cups basmati rice

2 tsp salt

½ cup finely chopped green onion

2 cups finely chopped dill

2 cups finely chopped parsley (leaves and fine stalks)

6 cups finely chopped cilantro (leaves and stalks)

3 tbsp grapeseed or another vegetable oil

1 small potato, peeled and very thinly sliced

3 tbsp water

1 cup Greek yogurt

½ cup sour cream

2 tbsp olive oil

Place the rice in a sieve and rinse thoroughly under running water. Transfer to a bowl and fill up with enough water to come ⅜ inch above the rice. Add the salt and stir. Leave to soak for 1 to 2 hours.

Take a large heavy pot and pour in the rice and its soaking liquid. Add more fresh water – about another 3 cups – to cover the rice well. Set on high heat and bring to the boil. Simmer for only a minute or so, then add the green onions and all the herbs and stir. Simmer for another 1 to 2 minutes, or until the rice just loses some of its hardness but is definitely not cooked yet. Drain in a sieve and set aside.

Rinse and dry the pot. Pour in 2 tablespoons of the oil and heat it over medium heat. Carefully arrange the potato slices, slightly overlapping, in the pan. Fry them, without stirring, for about 2 minutes, just to get a little color. Remove from the heat and allow to cool down.

Drizzle 2 tablespoons of the water over the potatoes, then start filling the pot with the rice. Do it gradually, using a large spoon, building up the rice into a proper heap on top of the potatoes and making sure as little rice as possible touches the sides of the pot.

Use the handle of a wooden spoon to make five deep holes in the rice, one in the center and four around it, all the way down to the potatoes. Turn the handle to carefully increase the diameter of each "chimney" to about ½ inch; these will assist the steaming.

Now drizzle the rice with the remaining 1 tablespoon each of grapeseed oil and water. Cover with a tight-fitting lid and leave on high heat for a minute or two, just to heat up. Reduce the heat to low and cook for 20 minutes. Turn off the heat and leave the rice, covered, to keep on steaming on the residual heat for another 20 minutes (if you have an electric stove, remove the pan from the burner to a warm place for the last 10 minutes).

Mix the yogurt with the sour cream. Fold in the olive oil without incorporating it fully. Serve over or next to the rice.

# Yogurt flatbreads with barley and mushrooms

This is a wonderfully soothing dish due to the smooth textures of the mushrooms and barley. As amazing as the flatbreads are, you don't have to make them if you are short of time. Rice or couscous will be fine alternatives.

Serves 6 as a starter

**Flatbreads**

1 cup plus 2 tsp whole-wheat flour

1½ tsp baking powder

½ tsp salt

¾ cup Greek yogurt

3 tbsp chopped fresh cilantro

4 tbsp clarified butter (or a mixture of melted butter and vegetable oil)

**Mushroom Ragout**

½ cup pearl barley

¾ oz dried porcini mushrooms

¾ cup lukewarm water

4 cups mixed shiitake and button mushrooms, halved

2 tbsp olive oil

5 tbsp butter

2 thyme sprigs

1 garlic clove, crushed

½ cup white wine

salt and black pepper

2 tbsp chopped parsley, plus extra to garnish

½ tbsp finely chopped preserved lemon

1 tbsp lemon juice

6 tbsp Greek yogurt

To make the flatbreads. Combine all the ingredients, apart from the butter, in a bowl and use your hands to mix them together to a dry dough; add more flour if needed. Knead the dough for a minute or so, until it is smooth and uniform. Wrap it in plastic wrap and chill for at least an hour.

To make the mushroom ragout. Rinse the barley with cold water, then place in a medium saucepan and cover with plenty of fresh water. Simmer for 30 to 35 minutes, or until al dente.

Place the porcini in a bowl and cover with lukewarm water; set aside. Put the fresh mushrooms in a heavy pan with the oil over medium-high heat, half the butter and the thyme, and sauté for 4 minutes, stirring occasionally. Once the mushrooms have softened, add the garlic and wine and allow to bubble away for about 5 minutes.

Next, add the porcini and their soaking liquid, leaving behind any grit in the bowl, plus some salt and pepper. Simmer on low heat for about 10 minutes. Finally, stir in the remaining butter with the parsley, preserved lemon, lemon juice and cooked barley. You will now have a flavorful mushroom stew with a thick sauce. Add more water if needed and taste for seasoning. Set aside; reheat before serving.

When ready to make the flatbreads, divide your dough into six pieces. Roll into balls, then flatten them with a rolling pin into round discs about 1 inch thick. Heat some clarified butter in a nonstick pan and fry the flatbreads, one at a time, on medium heat for about 2 minutes on each side, or until golden brown. Add more butter as you need it and keep the flatbreads warm as they are cooked.

To serve, fold each warm flatbread in half or into quarters and top with warm ragout, a spoonful of yogurt and a sprinkle of parsley.

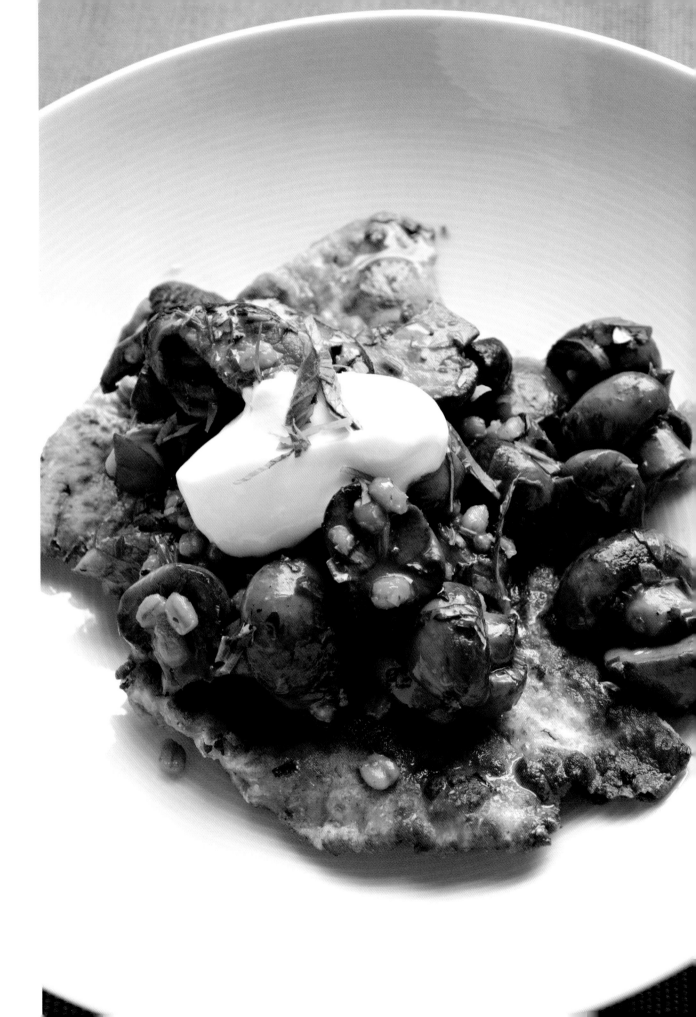

# Barley and pomegranate salad

You'll be surprised by how simple this salad is to make, considering how spectacular it tastes. I can almost promise that it is going to become a daily affair! It will go well with Fried Leeks (page 42) as well as many fatty cuts of meat.

Serves 4

1 cup pearl barley

6 celery stalks (leaves picked and
    reserved), cut into small dice

¼ cup olive oil

3 tbsp sherry vinegar

2 small garlic cloves, crushed

⅔ tsp ground allspice

salt and black pepper

3 tbsp chopped dill

3 tbsp chopped parsley

seeds from 2 large pomegranates
    (see page 110)

Rinse the barley with cold water, then place in a medium saucepan and cover with plenty of fresh water. Simmer for 30 to 35 minutes, or until tender but still with a bite.

Drain the barley and transfer to a mixing bowl. While it is still hot, add the celery, olive oil, vinegar, garlic, allspice and some salt and pepper. Stir, then leave to cool down completely.

Once cool, add the herbs, celery leaves and pomegranate seeds and mix in. Taste and adjust the seasoning to your liking, then serve.

# Kısır

This is my take on a classic Turkish dish that resonates with variations all over the Levant. Serve it with butter lettuce leaves as part of a mezze selection.

Serves 4

2 large onions, finely chopped

6 tbsp olive oil, plus extra to finish

2 tbsp tomato paste

4 medium tomatoes, peeled and chopped

½ cup water

1 cup medium bulgur wheat

1½ tsp pomegranate molasses

1 tbsp lemon juice

6 tbsp chopped parsley

3 green onions, finely shredded, plus extra to finish

2 fresh green chiles, seeded and finely chopped

2 garlic cloves, crushed

1 tsp ground cumin

salt and black pepper

seeds from 1 medium pomegranate (see page 110)

handful of mint leaves, some whole and some roughly shredded

Place the onions and olive oil in a large pan and sauté on medium heat for about 5 minutes, or until translucent. Add the tomato paste and stir with a wooden spoon for 2 minutes. Add the tomatoes and simmer on low heat for a further 4 minutes. Now add the water and bring to the boil. Remove immediately from the heat and stir in the bulgur.

Next, add the molasses, lemon juice, parsley, green onions, chiles, garlic, cumin and some salt and pepper. Stir well, then leave aside until the dish reaches room temperature or is just lukewarm. Taste it and adjust the seasoning; it will probably need plenty of salt.

Spoon the kısır onto serving dishes and flatten it out roughly with a spoon, creating a wave-like pattern on the surface. Scatter pomegranate seeds all over, drizzle with oil and finish with mint and green onion.

# Cardamom rice with poached eggs and yogurt

This is what you should cook on a late Sunday morning to really spoil your family. I can't get enough of it. Additions will be welcomed: consider peas, green beans, fried onions, buttered sunflower seeds and even golden raisins.

Serves 4

4 tbsp peanut oil, plus extra to finish
2 medium onions, finely chopped
4 garlic cloves, crushed
6 fresh curry leaves
8 cardamom pods
2 tsp coriander seeds
2 tsp ground turmeric
2 fresh green chiles, thinly sliced
coarse sea salt
2 cups basmati rice
3 cups plus 2 tbsp water
1 tbsp white wine vinegar
8 medium eggs
1⅓ cups parsley leaves, chopped
5 cups cilantro leaves, chopped
6 tbsp lime juice
8 tbsp Greek yogurt
black pepper

Preheat the oven to 350°F. Start with the rice. Heat up the peanut oil in a large, heavy, ovenproof saucepan for which you have a tight-fitting lid. Add the onions and garlic and sauté on low heat for 8 minutes. Add the curry leaves, cardamom, coriander seeds, turmeric, chiles and 1 teaspoon salt. Continue to cook and stir for 4 minutes on medium heat.

Add the rice and stir to coat in the oil. Add the water (it should come ⅜ inch above the rice). Cover the pan and put it into the oven. Cook for about 25 minutes. By this point the rice should be totally cooked. When you check, remove the lid very briefly so you don't lose all the steam in the pan. Remove the pan from the oven, keeping it covered, and set it aside somewhere warm.

Fill a shallow saucepan with enough water for a whole egg to cook in. Add the vinegar and bring to a rapid boil. Carefully break each egg into a cup, then gently pour into the boiling water. Immediately remove the pan from the heat and set it aside. After about 4 minutes the egg should be poached to perfection. Using a slotted spoon carefully transfer the poached egg to a bowl of warm water to keep it from cooling down. Once all the eggs are done, dry them on paper towels.

When you are nearly finished poaching the eggs, stir the parsley, cilantro and lime juice into the rice and fluff it up with a fork. Taste and adjust the seasoning.

Divide the rice among individual serving bowls and spoon yogurt on top. Place two eggs on each portion, drizzle some oil on top and sprinkle with salt and pepper.

# Freekeh pilaf

We normally enjoy grains once they have matured and dried, but there is a widespread culinary tradition of consuming green, semi-mature grains, which taste grassier and are more nutritious than the dried version. Throughout the Middle East it is common to process young and green durum wheat into freekeh. This is done by literally burning the wheat head in order to scorch the chaff and thus to assist removing the grain. The result is lightly charred green grains with a wonderful smoky aroma, which are often used like rice or bulgur wheat. Freekeh isn't easy to find but you should come across it in Middle Eastern grocery shops. Or you can use bulgur as a substitute, in which case reduce the cooking time by 10 minutes and leave to stand as with the freekeh.

The key to this dish is good stock with a lot of flavor. As Arabs normally cook freekeh in chicken or mutton stock, I suggest reducing a good vegetable stock by half to intensify it.

Serves 2–4
2 medium onions, thinly sliced
2 tbsp butter
1 tbsp olive oil, plus extra to finish
1 cup freekeh (or bulgur wheat)
¼ tsp ground cinnamon
¼ tsp ground allspice
1¼ cups good-quality reduced vegetable stock
salt and black pepper
½ cup Greek yogurt
1½ tsp lemon juice
½ garlic clove, crushed
⅛ cup finely chopped parsley, plus extra to garnish
⅛ cup finely chopped mint
⅔ cup finely chopped cilantro
2 tbsp pine nuts, toasted and roughly broken

Place the onions, butter and olive oil in a large heavy pot and sauté on a medium heat, stirring occasionally, for 15 to 20 minutes, or until the onion is soft and brown.

Meanwhile, soak the freekeh in cold water for 5 minutes. Drain in a sieve and rinse well under cold running water. Drain well.

Add the freekeh and spices to the onions, followed by the stock and some salt and pepper. Stir well. Bring to the boil, then cover, reduce the heat to a bare minimum and leave to simmer for 15 minutes. Remove the pan from the heat and leave it covered for 5 minutes. Finally, remove the lid and leave the pilaf to cool down a little, about another 5 minutes.

While you wait, mix the yogurt with the lemon juice, garlic and some salt.

Stir the herbs into the warm (not hot) pilaf. Taste and adjust the seasoning. Spoon onto serving dishes and top each portion with a generous dollop of yogurt. Sprinkle with pine nuts and parsley and finish with a trickle of olive oil.

# Itamar's bulgur pilaf

Full of little surprises – whole pink peppercorns, currants, coriander seeds – this is one of the most comforting dishes I've come across. You can serve it with Leek Fritters (page 36) and their sauce to create a light meal from heaven, or next to Smoky Frittata (page 96) with some Greek yogurt on the side. A million thank-yous to Itamar Srulovich.

Serves 4–6
about 6 tbsp olive oil
4 small white onions, thinly sliced
3 red bell peppers, cut into thin strips
2½ tbsp tomato paste
1 tbsp sugar
2 tsp pink peppercorns
2 tbsp coriander seeds
⅔ cup currants
1 cup medium bulgur wheat
1¾ cups water
salt and black pepper
handful of chopped chives

Heat up the olive oil in a large pot and sauté the onions and peppers together over medium–high heat for 12 to 15 minutes, or until they soften up completely.

Next, add the tomato paste, sugar, spices and currants and stir as you cook for about 2 minutes. Add the bulgur, water, and some salt and pepper. Stir to mix, then bring to the boil. As soon as the water boils, cover the pot with a tight-fitting lid, remove from the heat and leave to sit for at least 20 minutes.

Finally, fluff up the bulgur with a fork and stir in the chives. If the pilaf seems dry, add a little more olive oil. Taste and adjust the seasoning; it's likely to need more salt and pepper. Serve warm.

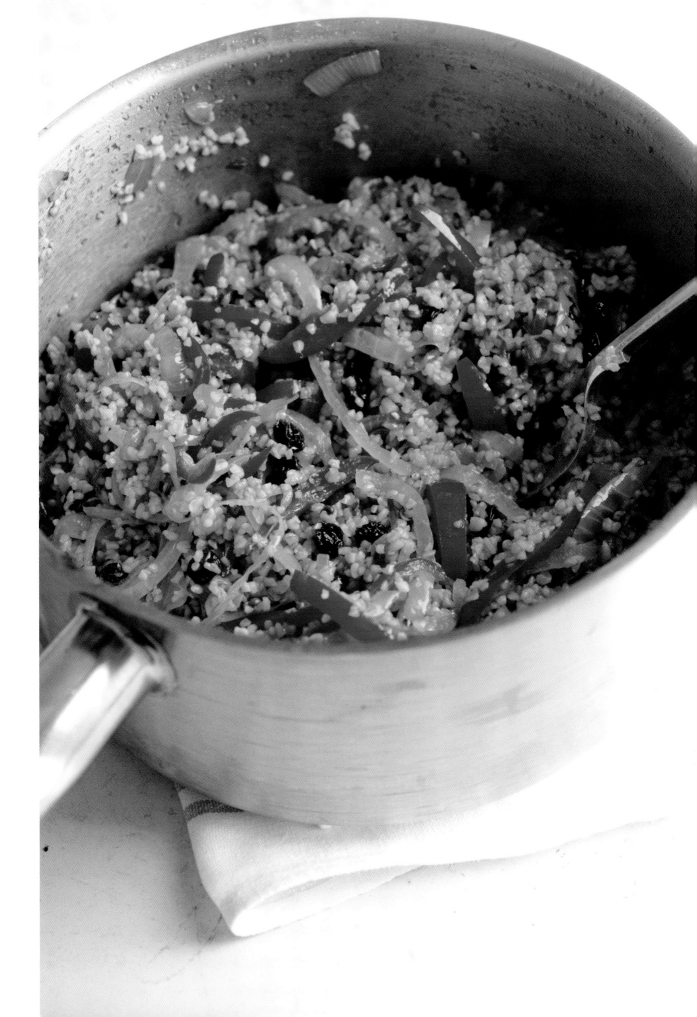

# Mango and coconut rice salad

Everybody knows now that the undisputed king of mangoes is the Indian Alphonso. It is intensely sweet and has an unbeatable perfumed aroma. I'd go as far as saying that you haven't tasted a real mango until you've tried an Alphonso (and nobody is paying me for this). The season, though, is very short – mid-April to the end of May – so try to prepare this salad (pictured on page 246) then.

Serves 4

⅔ cup jasmine or basmati rice

1 tsp unsalted butter

salt

½ cup water

1 cup loosely packed Thai basil

1 cup Camargue red rice

1 red bell pepper, thinly sliced

2 tbsp mint leaves, roughly chopped

⅔ cup cilantro leaves, roughly chopped

2 green onions, thinly sliced

1 fresh red chile, seeded and finely chopped

grated zest and juice of 1 lemon

1 large mango or 2 smaller ones, cut roughly into 1-inch dice

½ cup roasted salted peanuts, roughly chopped

⅔ cup flaked coconut

2 tbsp peanut oil

¾ cup crisp-fried shallots (homemade or bought, optional)

Start by cooking the rice. Put the jasmine rice and butter in a small saucepan and place on a medium heat. Add a little salt, the water and half the Thai basil (keep the leaves attached to the stalk). Bring to the boil, then cover and cook on a slow simmer for 15 to 20 minutes. Remove and discard the basil. Spread out the rice on a flat tray to cool down.

Cook the red rice in plenty of boiling water (as you would cook pasta but with no salt) for 20 minutes, or until it is cooked through. Drain and spread on a tray to cool down.

Pick off the leaves of the remaining basil and chop them up roughly. Place them in a large mixing bowl. Add the jasmine and red rice together with all the remaining ingredients, apart from the shallots, and stir just to mix; do not stir too much or the mango pieces will disintegrate. Taste and adjust the seasoning. Transfer the salad into serving bowls and garnish with crisp-fried shallots, if you like.

# Quinoa salad with dried Persian lime

I recently started using a new addictive substance – the small dried limes (or lemons) that appear widely in Iranian cooking. They add a fantastic sharpness and unique perfumed aroma to stews and marinades. For long-cooked wet dishes you just throw one in, lightly perforated, and it will impart its flavor to the whole dish. In this salad (pictured on page 247), though, I use it in powdered form. Unfortunately this is not simple to achieve because the limes are rock hard. If you have a spice grinder you should be fine; however, a food processor will struggle and give you some powder that you'll then need to sieve. You can buy the limes in powder form but this is not as potent as what you make yourself. You can find dried limes online at kalustyans.com and from most Middle Eastern and North African shops.

Serves 4–6
2 medium sweet potatoes (about 12 oz each)
7 tbsp olive oil
salt and black pepper
1 cup mixed basmati and wild rice
1 cup quinoa
4 garlic cloves, thinly sliced
3 tbsp shredded sage leaves
3 tbsp roughly chopped oregano
2 tbsp ground dried Persian lime
6 tbsp shredded mint
4 green onions (green parts only), thinly sliced, plus extra to finish
1 tsp lemon juice
6 oz feta, crumbled

Preheat the oven to 400°F. Peel the sweet potatoes and cut them into roughly 1-inch dice. Spread in a baking pan lined with parchment paper, drizzle over half the oil and sprinkle with salt and pepper. Roast for 20 to 25 minutes, or until tender.

Meanwhile, cook the basmati and wild rice as instructed on the packet; drain. Place the quinoa in a pan with plenty of boiling water and simmer for 9 minutes; drain in a fine sieve. When dry (but still warm), transfer the rice and quinoa to a large mixing bowl.

Pour the remaining oil into a small frying pan to heat up, then fry the garlic for about 30 seconds, or until it turns light golden. Add the sage and oregano and stir as you fry for about a minute; watch to be sure that the herbs or garlic don't burn. Pour the contents of the pan over the rice and quinoa.

Next, add the roasted sweet potato with its oil. Add the lime powder, mint, green onions, lemon juice, feta, and some salt and pepper. Toss everything together gently, being careful not to mush up the sweet potato and feta. Taste and adjust the seasoning. Serve warmish, or at room temperature, garnished with green onions.

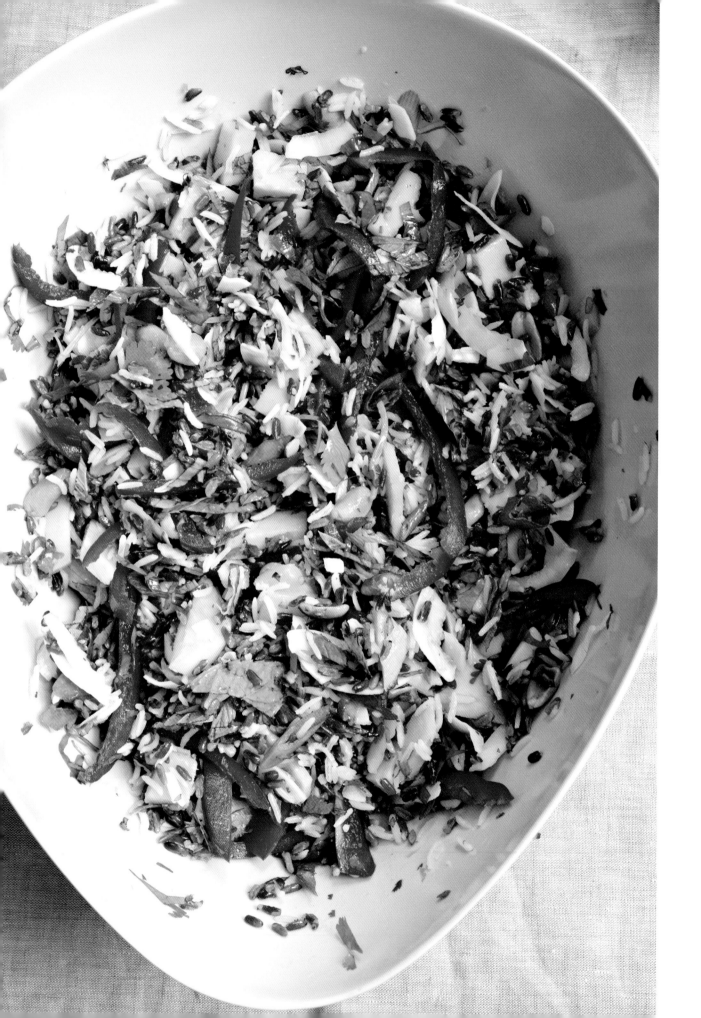

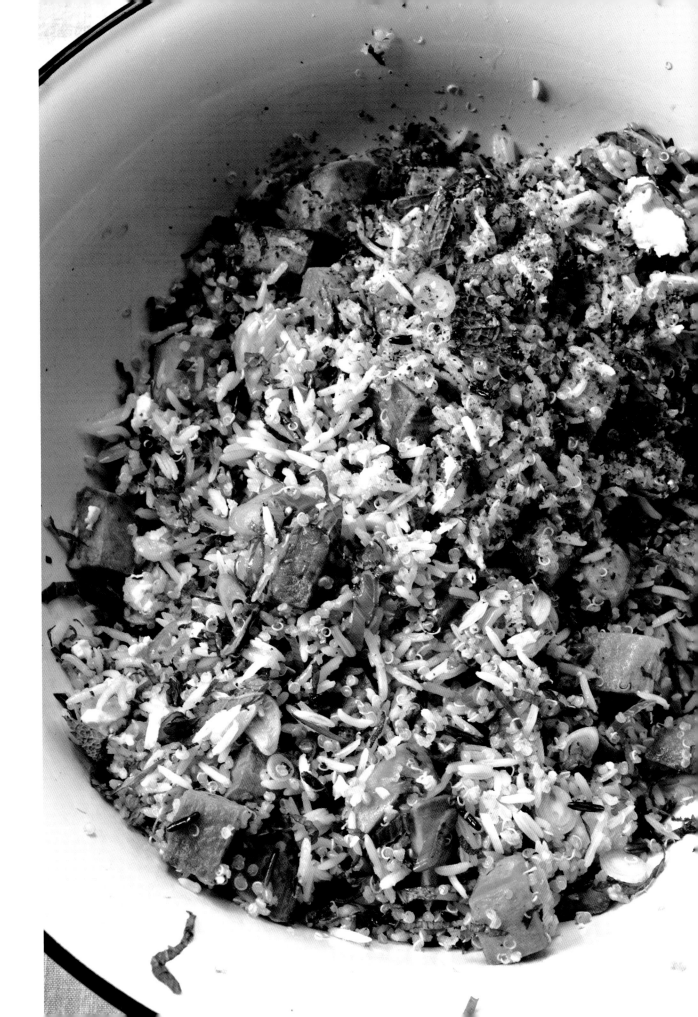

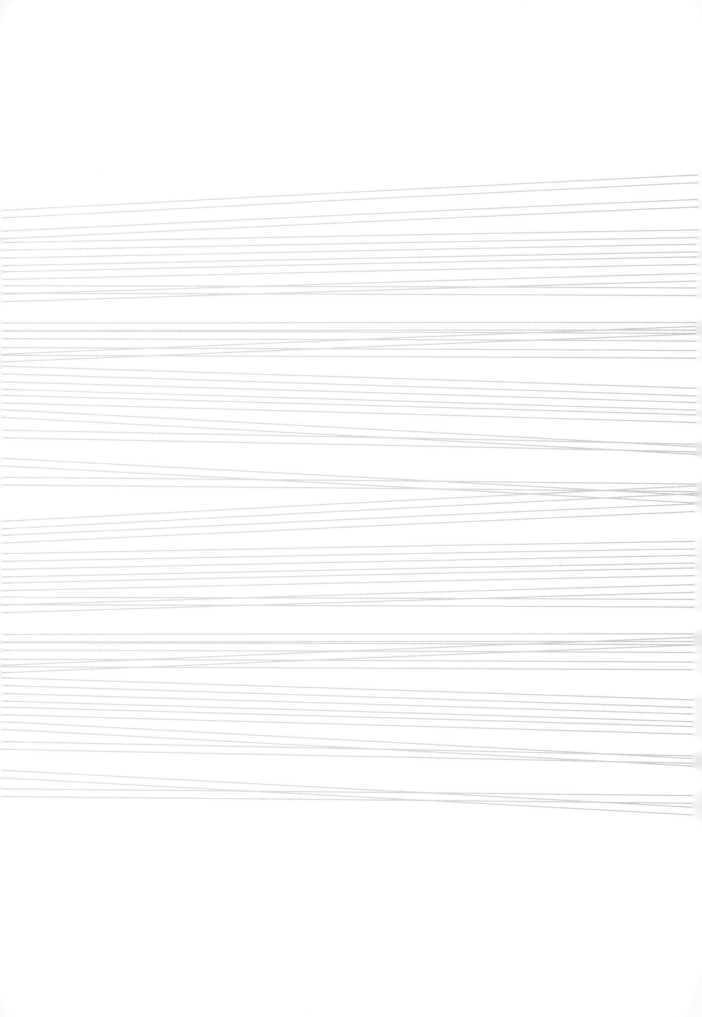

Pasta, Polenta, Couscous

# Lemon and goat cheese ravioli

The trade-off for having to make your own pasta here is that there's no sauce to labor over. The combination of melting cheese, grapeseed oil and pink peppercorns is delicate yet clearly present and satisfying. Choose a relatively soft and quite mild goat cheese.

Serves 4 as a starter

**Pasta dough**

3 tbsp olive oil

3 medium eggs

11½ oz (about 2¾ cups) "00" pasta flour, plus extra for rolling

¼ tsp ground turmeric

grated zest of 3 lemons

semolina

**Filling**

11 oz soft goat cheese

⅓ tsp Maldon sea salt

pinch of chile flakes

black pepper

1 egg white, beaten

2 tsp pink peppercorns, finely crushed

1 tsp chopped tarragon

grated zest of 1 lemon

grapeseed oil

lemon juice (optional)

To make the pasta dough. Whisk together the oil and eggs. Put the flour, turmeric and lemon zest in a food processor, add the oil and egg mixture and blend to a crumbly dough. It might require extra flour or oil. Once the dough has come together and is smooth (you may need to work it a little by hand), divide it into four thick, rectangular blocks. Wrap them in plastic wrap and chill for at least 30 minutes, or up to 2 days.

Lightly dust a work surface with flour. Take one piece of dough and flatten it on the floured surface with a rolling pin. Set your pasta machine to the widest setting and pass the dough through. Repeat, narrowing the setting by a notch each time, until you get to the lowest setting. When each sheet is rolled, keep it under a moist towel so it doesn't dry out.

To make the filling. Combine the filling ingredients, apart from the egg white, in a bowl and crush together with a fork.

Use a pastry cutter or the rim of a glass to stamp out roughly 3-inch discs from the pasta sheets. To shape each raviolo, brush a disc with a little egg white and place a heaped teaspoon of filling in its center. Place another pasta disc on top. Dip your fingers in flour, then gently press out any air as you seal the edges of the two discs together. You should end up with a pillow-shaped center surrounded by an edge that is just under ⅜ inch wide. Seal the sides of the edges together firmly until you can't see a seam where the two discs meet. As they are made, place the ravioli on a dish towel or tray sprinkled with semolina. Leave to dry for 10 to 15 minutes. (You can now cover the tray with plastic wrap and keep the ravioli in the fridge for a day.)

When ready to cook, bring a large pan of salted water to the boil. Cook the pasta for 2 to 3 minutes, or until al dente. Drain and divide among four plates. Sprinkle with pink peppercorns, tarragon and lemon zest. Drizzle grapeseed oil over the ravioli and around them, sprinkle with extra salt and a squirt of lemon juice, if you like, and serve at once.

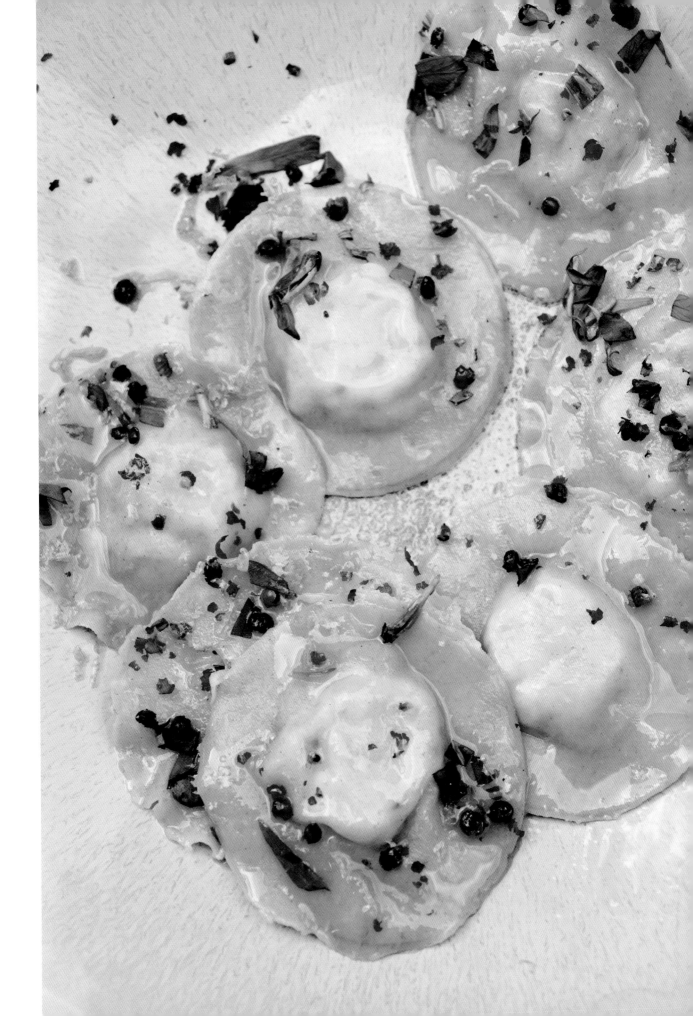

# Crunchy pappardelle

I use panko, the crisp Japanese breadcrumbs, to add texture to this creamy pasta. The sauce dries out easily so I add some of the pasta's cooking liquid before serving; make sure it is quite runny.

Serves 2

¼ cup olive oil

3½ cups button mushrooms, halved

7 tbsp white wine

1 bay leaf

3 thyme sprigs, leaves picked and chopped

½ tsp sugar

⅔ cup heavy cream

salt and black pepper

grated zest of 1 lemon

1 garlic clove, crushed

3 tbsp chopped parsley

3 tbsp panko

1 bunch broccolini

9 oz dried pappardelle

Bring a large pot of salted water and a small pot of salted water to a boil. Heat the olive oil over medium-high heat in a large saucepan and sauté the mushrooms until they start taking on color, stirring occasionally. Add the wine, bay leaf, thyme and sugar. Bring to the boil and reduce the liquid by two-thirds. Add the cream and stir to mix. Taste and add plenty of salt and pepper. Keep warm.

Mix together the lemon zest, garlic and parsley. In a pan over medium heat, toast the panko until golden, stirring occasionally.

Pick any leaves from the broccolini, then cut into 2½-inch-long pieces (stalks and florets). If the stalks are thick, cut them along the center in half or into quarters. Blanch in the small pot of boiling water for 2 minutes and drain.

Add the pasta to the large pot of boiling water. When the pasta is just ready, add the broccolini to the cream sauce to reheat. Drain the pappardelle, keeping some of the cooking liquid, and stir with the cream sauce; add half of the parsley mix. If the sauce seems dry, add some of the reserved cooking liquid.

Transfer the pasta to a serving bowl. Stir the rest of the parsley mix into the panko and sprinkle generously over the pappardelle, then serve immediately.

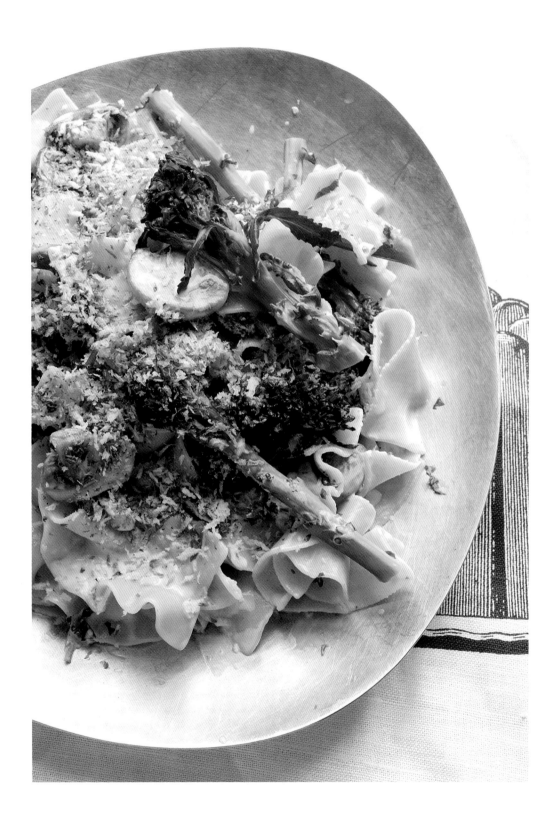

# Pasta and fried zucchini salad

I put to good use here my grandmother's fried zucchini, her signature Passover dish. They are as beautiful on their own as they are in this salad (pictured on page 256), which makes ideal picnic grub. The pasta I've used is *strozzapreti*, which literally means "priest choker"! Feel free to substitute another interesting short pasta shape.

Serves 4
²⁄₃ cup sunflower oil
3 medium zucchini, cut into ¼-inch-thick slices
1½ tbsp red wine vinegar
¾ cup frozen edamame
2 cups basil leaves, shredded coarsely
¼ cup parsley leaves
⅓ cup olive oil
salt and black pepper
9 oz  strozzapreti or penne
grated zest of 1 lemon
1½ tbsp small capers
7 oz buffalo mozzarella, torn by hand into chunks

Bring a large pot of salted water to a boil. Heat the sunflower oil in a medium saucepan over medium-high heat. Fry the zucchini slices in a few batches, making sure you don't crowd them, for 3 minutes, or until golden brown on both sides; turn them over once only. As they are cooked, transfer to a colander to drain. Tip the zucchini slices into a bowl, pour over the vinegar and stir, then set aside.

Blanch the edamame for 3 minutes in boiling water; drain, refresh under running cold water and set aside to dry.

Combine half the basil, all of the parsley and the olive oil in a food processor, adding a bit of salt and pepper. Blitz to a smooth sauce.

Cook the pasta until al dente; drain and rinse under a stream of cold water. Return to the pan in which it was cooked.

Pour the zucchini and their juices over the pasta. Add the edamame, basil sauce, lemon zest, capers and mozzarella. Stir gently together, then taste and season with plenty of salt and pepper. Before serving, stir in the remaining basil.

# Green couscous

A good-looking and even better tasting side salad (pictured on page 257). It has strong flavors and is extremely healthful but still feels light and comforting. Serve it with Poached Baby Vegetables (page 12) or with fish. Adding some feta will make it a bit more substantial.

Serves 4
1 cup couscous
¾ cup boiling water or vegetable stock
1 small onion, thinly sliced
1 tbsp olive oil
¼ tsp salt
¼ tsp ground cumin

Herb paste
⅓ cup chopped parsley
1 cup chopped cilantro
2 tbsp chopped tarragon
2 tbsp chopped dill
2 tbsp chopped mint
6 tbsp olive oil

½ cup unsalted pistachios, toasted and
    roughly chopped
3 green onions, finely sliced
1 fresh green chile, finely sliced
1¼ cup arugula leaves, chopped

Place the couscous in a large bowl and cover with the boiling water or stock. Cover the bowl with plastic wrap and leave for 10 minutes.

Meanwhile, fry the onion in the olive oil on medium heat until golden and completely soft. Add the salt and cumin and mix well. Leave to cool slightly.

To make the herb paste. Place all the ingredients in a food processor and blitz until smooth.

Add the herb paste to the couscous and mix everything together well with a fork to fluff it up. Now add the cooked onion, the pistachios, green onions, green chile and arugula and gently mix. Serve at room temperature.

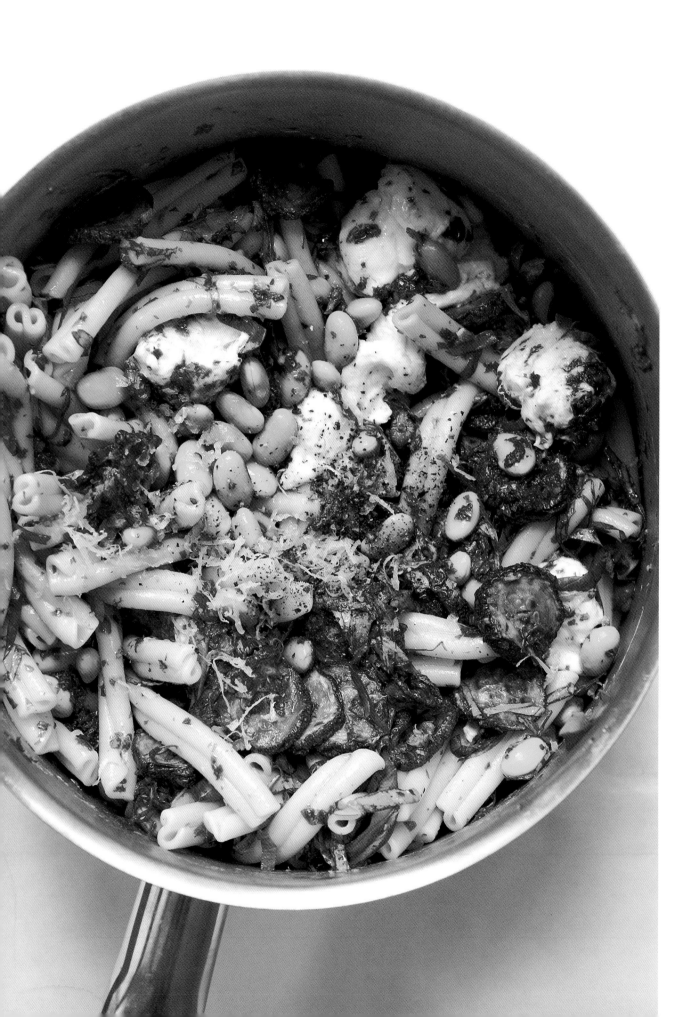

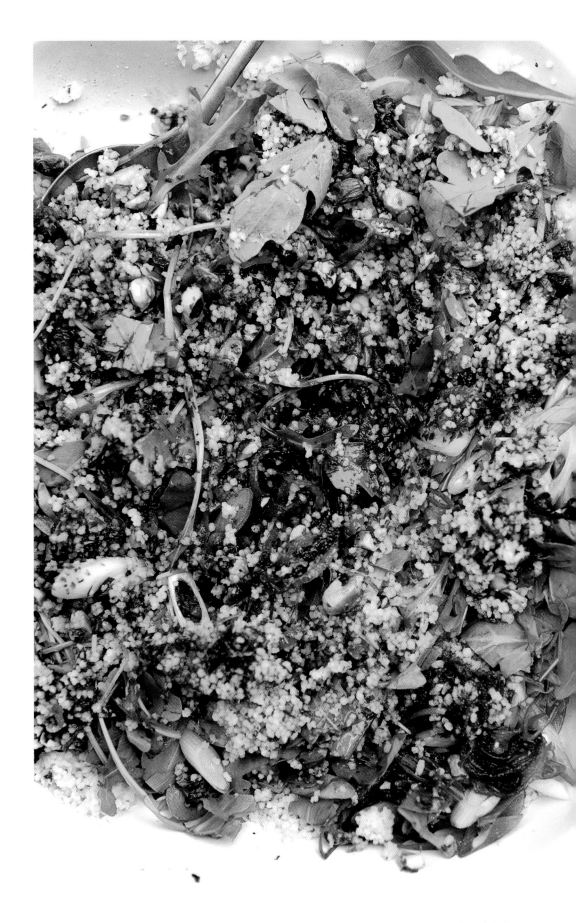

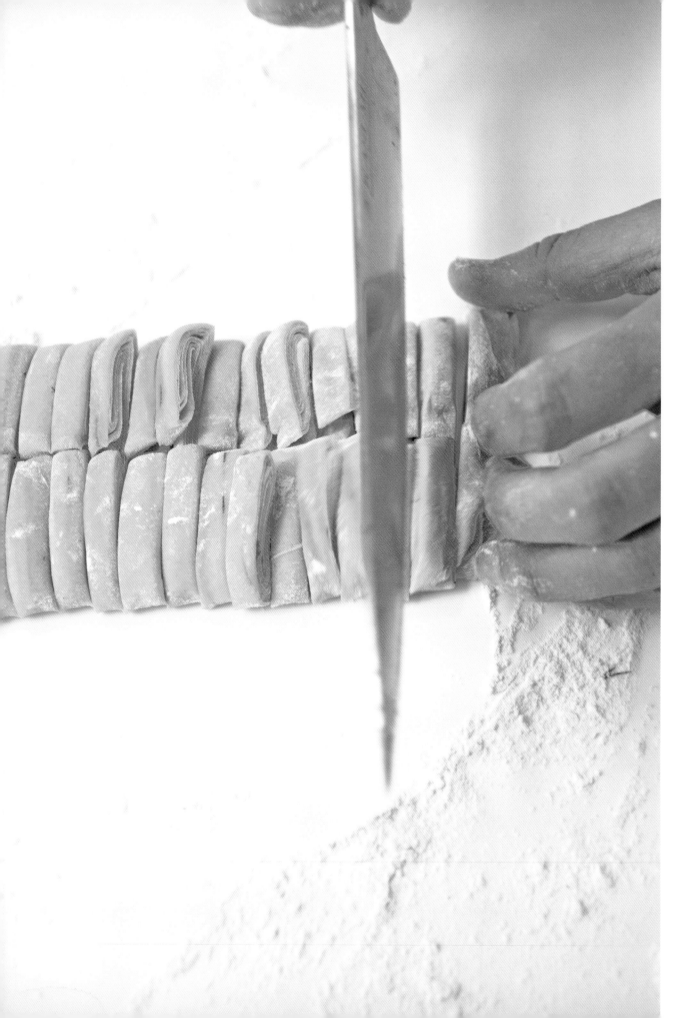

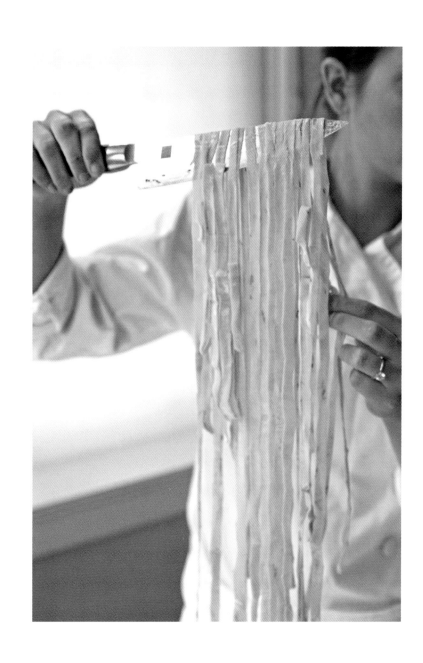

# Saffron tagliatelle with spiced butter

Counterintuitive as this combination of pasta with Moroccan-style butter may seem, it is absolutely delicious and I am sure that once tried you'll keep on coming back to it. Instead of homemade you can go for a good variety of dried pasta and add a decent pinch of saffron threads to the cooking water.

Serves 4
2 tsp saffron threads
4 tbsp boiling water
4 medium eggs
4 tbsp olive oil
15½ oz (3½ cups) "00" pasta flour, plus extra for rolling
1 tsp ground turmeric

Spiced butter
1 cup (2 sticks) butter
4 tbsp olive oil
8 shallots, finely chopped
1 tsp ground ginger
1 tsp sweet paprika
1 tsp ground coriander
1 tsp ground cinnamon
1 tsp cayenne pepper
½ tsp chile flakes
½ tsp ground turmeric
1 tsp salt
black pepper

⅔ cup pine nuts, toasted and roughly chopped
4 tbsp roughly chopped mint
4 tbsp roughly chopped parsley

Place the saffron in a small bowl with the boiling water and leave to infuse for at least 10 minutes. Then add the eggs and oil and beat to mix. Place the flour and turmeric in the bowl of a food processor and add the saffron mix. Blend until a crumbly dough is formed. You may need a little more oil or flour to adjust the dough to the required consistency – neither sticky nor very dry.

Lightly dust your surface with flour, tip out the dough and knead into a ball. Work for a few minutes, adding more flour if you need, until it becomes silky soft. Wrap the dough in plastic wrap and chill for 30 minutes, or up to a day.

Divide the dough into two pieces. Keep one well covered. Using a rolling pin, flatten the other piece into a thin rectangle. Set the pasta machine to its widest setting and pass the dough through. Continue rolling the pasta, narrowing the setting by a notch every time, until you get to the lowest setting.

Fold up the pasta sheet twice along its length, sprinkling some flour between the layers. Use a large knife to cut long strips that are ¾ inch wide. Hang them on the back of a chair to dry for 10 minutes. Repeat with the remaining dough.

Bring a large pot of salted water to a boil.

To make the spiced butter. Place the butter and oil in a frying pan and cook the shallots gently for about 10 minutes, or until they soften and the butter turns slightly brown. Now add all the spices, the salt and some pepper. Remove from the heat and keep warm.

Cook the tagliatelle for 2 to 3 minutes, or until al dente. Drain and return to the saucepan. Pour the spiced butter over the pasta and stir well, then divide among four plates. Sprinkle with the pine nuts and chopped herbs and serve.

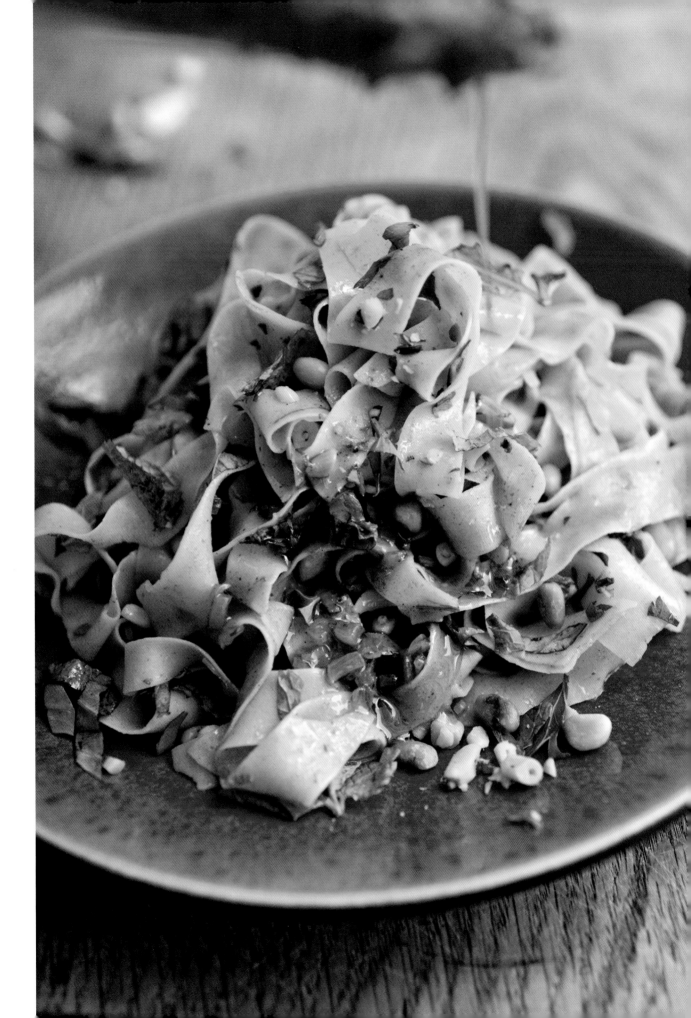

# The ultimate winter couscous

Someone complained to the *Guardian* about the long list of ingredients in this recipe. But I knew it was a success when a friend spotted it on the menu (with a due credit) of the Sun and Doves, a cool and arty pub in Camberwell.

Serves 4, or even more

2 medium carrots, peeled and cut into
  ¾-inch chunks

2 medium parsnips, peeled and cut into
  ¾-inch chunks

8 shallots, peeled

2 cinnamon sticks

4 star anise

3 bay leaves

5 tbsp olive oil

salt

½ tsp ground ginger

¼ tsp ground turmeric

¼ tsp hot paprika

¼ tsp chile flakes

2½ cups cubed pumpkin or butternut
  squash (from a 10 oz squash)

½ cup dried apricots, roughly chopped

1 cup chickpeas (canned or freshly
  cooked)

1½ cups chickpea cooking liquid and/
  or water

1 cup couscous

large pinch of saffron

1 cup boiling vegetable stock

3 tbsp butter, broken into pieces

2 tbsp harissa

1 oz preserved lemon, finely chopped

2 cups cilantro leaves

Preheat the oven to 375°F. Place the carrots, parsnips and shallots in a large ovenproof dish. Add the cinnamon sticks, star anise, bay leaves, 4 tablespoons of the oil, ¾ teaspoon salt and all the other spices and mix well. Place in the oven and cook for 15 minutes.

Add the pumpkin, stir and return to the oven. Continue cooking for about 35 minutes, by which time the vegetables should have softened while retaining a bite. Now add the dried apricots and the chickpeas with their cooking liquid and/or water. Return to the oven and cook for a further 10 minutes, or until hot.

About 15 minutes before the vegetables are ready, put the couscous in a large heatproof bowl with the remaining 1 tablespoon olive oil, the saffron and ½ teaspoon salt. Pour the boiling stock over the couscous. Cover the bowl with plastic wrap and leave for about 10 minutes. Then add the butter and fluff up the couscous with a fork until the butter melts in. Cover again and leave somewhere warm.

To serve, spoon couscous into a deep plate or bowl. Stir the harissa and preserved lemon into the vegetables; taste and add salt if needed. Spoon the vegetables onto the center of the couscous. Finish with plenty of cilantro leaves.

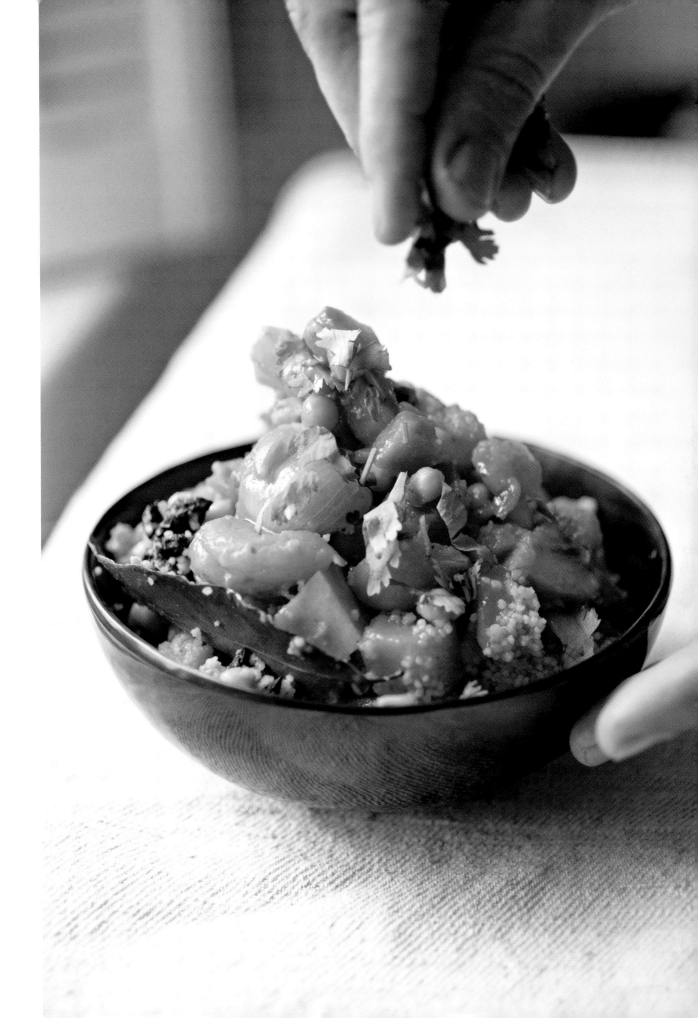

# Mushroom and herb polenta

When cooking polenta my father always makes much more than he needs. Half of it he serves right away in the runny state, like a mash, with a flavorful sauce. The rest he spreads onto an oiled surface and allows to set. The next day he cuts out chunks, fries them in olive oil and serves with a chunky vegetable salad (tomato, cucumber, romaine lettuce) dressed lightly with red wine vinegar and olive oil. The dish here uses soft polenta, but you may want to double the quantity to follow my father's idea.

Note that there are two types of polenta meal (or cornmeal) available – a quick or instant variety and the traditional, slow-cooking one. For most purposes I find that the quick polenta is good enough. Either one can be used for this dish.

Serves 2
4 tbsp olive oil
4 cups mixed mushrooms, very large ones halved
2 garlic cloves, crushed
1 tablespoon chopped tarragon
1 tablespoon chopped thyme
1 tablespoon truffle oil
salt and black pepper
2¼ cups vegetable stock
½ cup polenta (instant or traditional)
3 oz Parmesan, grated
2½ tbsp butter
1 teaspoon finely chopped rosemary
1 tablespoon chopped chervil
4 oz Taleggio (rind removed), cut into ⅜-inch slices

Heat half the olive oil in a large frying pan over medium-high heat. Once hot, add half of the mushrooms and fry for a few minutes, or until just cooked; try not to move them much so you get golden-brown patches on their surface. Remove from the pan, and repeat with the rest of the mushrooms and oil. Off the heat, return all the mushrooms to the pan and add the garlic, tarragon, thyme, truffle oil and some salt and pepper. Keep warm.

Bring the stock to the boil in a saucepan. Slowly stir in the polenta, then reduce the heat to the minimum and cook, stirring constantly with a wooden spoon. The polenta is ready when it leaves the sides of the pan but is still runny. If you are using instant polenta this shouldn't take more than 5 minutes; with traditional polenta it could take up to 50 minutes (if it seems to dry out, add some more stock or water but just enough to keep it at a thick porridge consistency).

Preheat the broiler. When the polenta is ready, stir in the Parmesan, butter, rosemary and half the chervil. Season with salt and pepper. Spread the polenta over a heatproof dish and top with the Taleggio. Place under the broiler until the cheese bubbles. Remove, top with the mushrooms and their juices, and return to the broiler for a minute to warm up. Serve hot, garnished with the remaining chervil.

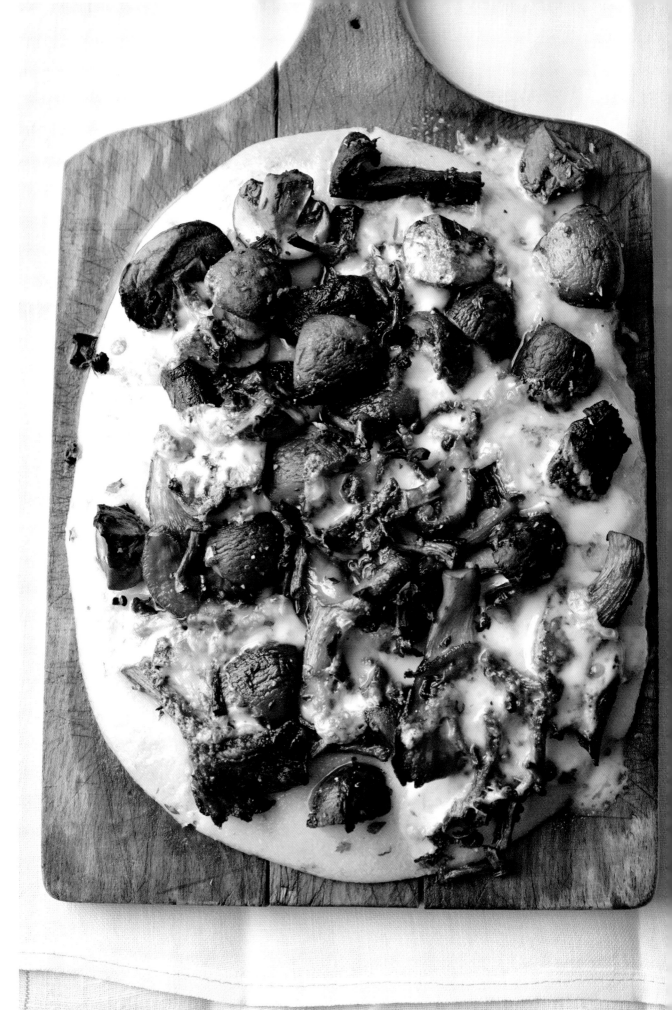

# Sweet corn polenta

Polenta made from fresh corn is almost like baby food, but in a good sense. It is smooth, sweet and soothing, a bit like a chunky savory porridge. It is my ideal heartwarming supper meal. Just keep in mind that it is nothing like regular polenta made from cornmeal – it is softer and not as substantial.

This dish (pictured on pages 268 and 269) is a variation on a recipe by two inspiring Israeli food writers, Haim Cohen and Eli Landau.

Serves 4

**Eggplant sauce**
⅔ cup vegetable oil
1 medium eggplant, cut into ¾-inch dice
2 tsp tomato paste
¼ cup white wine
1 cup chopped peeled tomatoes (fresh or canned)
6½ tbsp water
¼ tsp salt
¼ tsp sugar
1 tbsp chopped oregano

**Polenta**
6 ears of corn
2¼ cups water
3 tbsp butter, diced
7 oz feta, crumbled
¼ tsp salt
black pepper

To make the eggplant sauce. Heat up the oil in a large saucepan and fry the eggplant on medium heat for about 15 minutes, or until nicely brown. Drain off as much oil as you can and discard it. Add the tomato paste to the pan and stir with the eggplant. Cook for 2 minutes, then add the wine and cook for 1 minute. Add the chopped tomatoes, water, salt, sugar and oregano and cook for a further 5 minutes to get a deep-flavored sauce. Set aside; warm it up when needed.

To make the polenta. Remove the leaves and "silk" from each ear of corn, then chop off the pointed top and stalk. Stand each ear upright on its base and use a sharp knife to shave off the kernels. You want to have 1¼ lbs of kernels.

Place the kernels in a medium saucepan and cover them with the water. Cook for 12 minutes on a low simmer. Use a slotted spoon to lift the kernels from the water and into a food processor; reserve the cooking liquid. Process them for quite a few minutes, to break as much of the kernel case as possible. Add some of the cooking liquid if the mixture becomes too dry to process.

Now return the corn paste to the pan with the cooking liquid and cook, while stirring, on low heat for 10 to 15 minutes, or until the mixture thickens to a mashed potato consistency. Fold in the butter, the feta, salt and some pepper and cook for a further 2 minutes. Taste and add more salt if needed.

Divide the polenta among shallow bowls and spoon some warm eggplant sauce in the center.

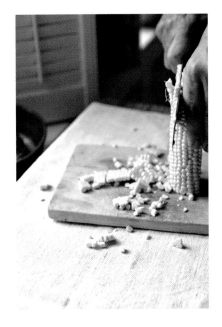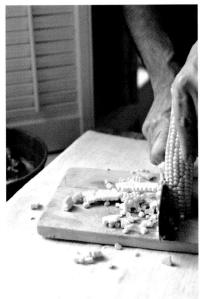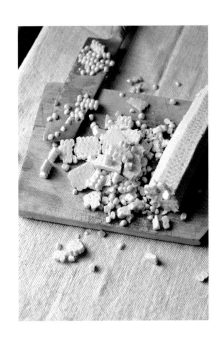

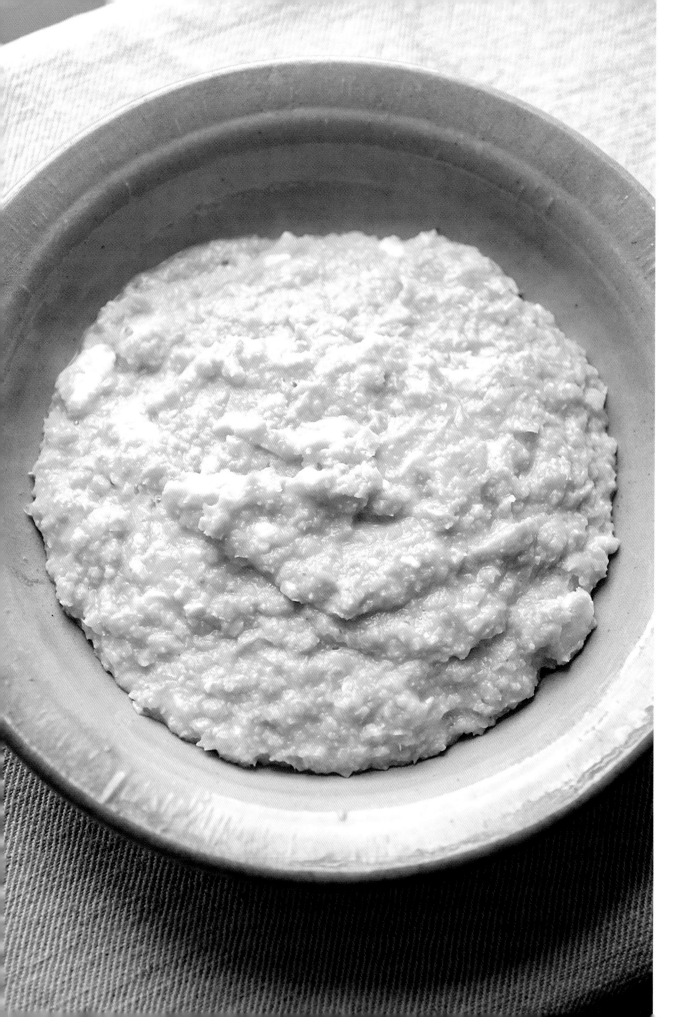

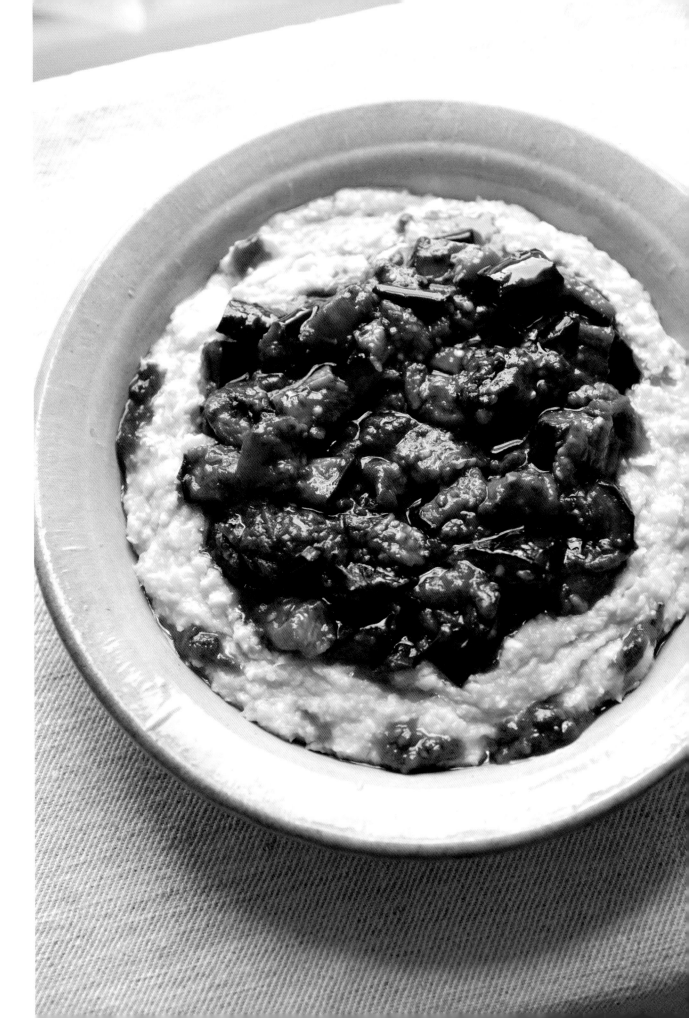

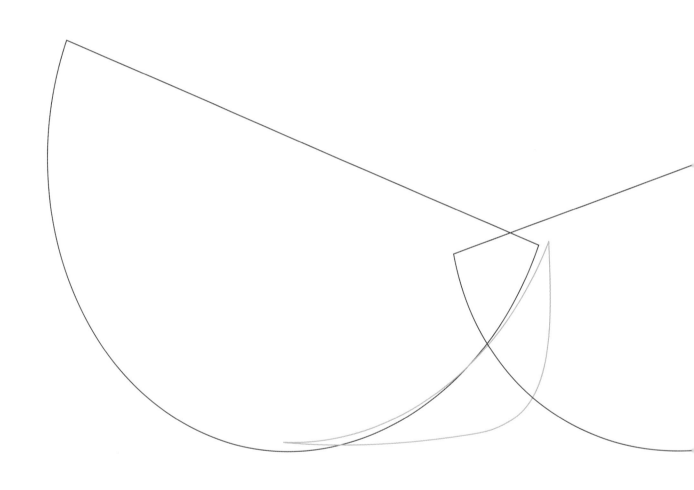

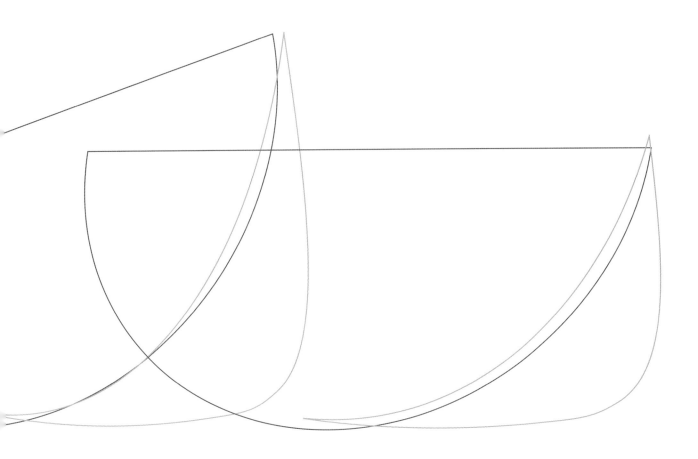

Fruit with Cheese

# Figs with basil, goat cheese and pomegranate vinaigrette

Fresh figs are available in summer and then make another short appearance in autumn. When they are good they are amazing, a word I use way too often, although in this case I totally stand behind it. The unctuous sweetness of a fresh fig, combined with its ripe-rich texture, is unbeatable. In Israel and Palestine fig trees are to be found everywhere, and picking the fruit and eating it straight off the tree is a childhood experience I am afraid I can't replicate in the United Kingdom. Still, I can buy good French or Italian figs, a day or two old, from La Fromagerie in London. Good figs are heavy and slightly squidgy and have a noticeable sweet smell; they often tend to crack at their base. Stick to those and you'll be fine. But no matter what you do, don't buy under-ripe supermarket figs that have been cargoed here from the ends of the world. Use a very young and creamy goat cheese (see Caramelized Fennel with Goat Cheese, page 172).

Serves 4
1 shallot, finely chopped
½ tsp Dijon mustard
2 tsp pomegranate molasses
salt and black pepper
3 tbsp olive oil, plus extra to finish
1½ cups arugula
¾ cup mixed purple and green basil
    leaves
8 ripe figs, at room temperature
2½ oz young and creamy goat cheese

Place the shallot, mustard and pomegranate molasses in a medium bowl. Add some salt and pepper and whisk vigorously as you slowly pour in the olive oil. You are aiming for a homogenous dressing.

Add most of the arugula and basil leaves to the dressing, reserving some to finish the salad, and toss gently. Lift the dressed leaves onto a large serving plate, spreading them out to line it.

Cut the figs vertically into quarters and arrange over the leaves. Next, dot the figs and leaves with teaspoonfuls of cheese. Scatter the reserved leaves on top, drizzle with extra oil and season with some salt and pepper.

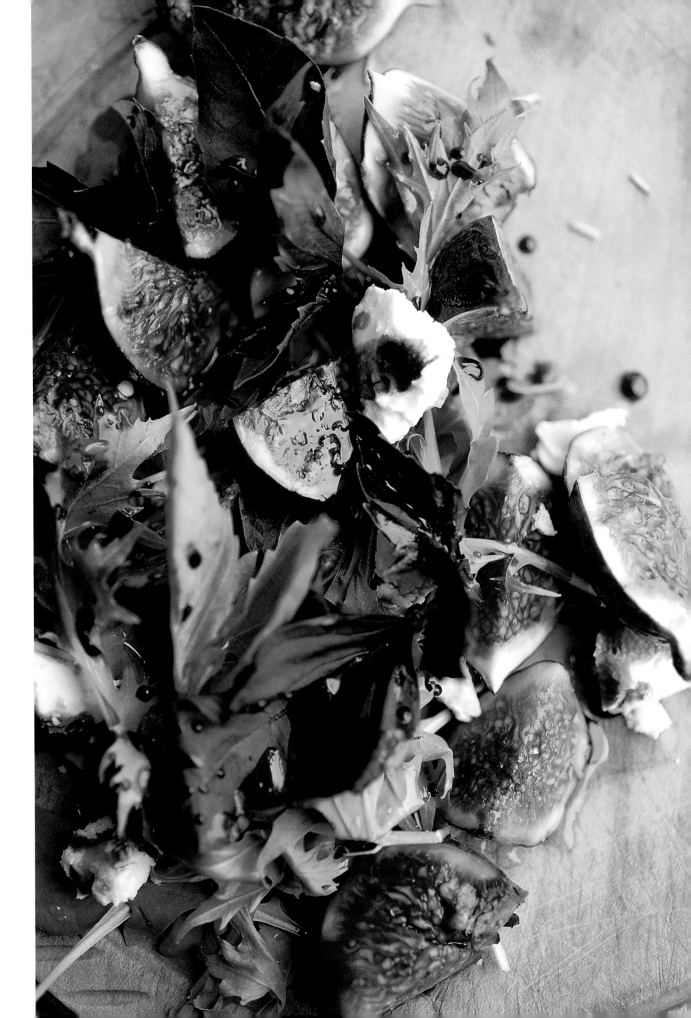

# Goat cheese soufflés with vanilla-poached peaches

Back in the 1990s I was the pastry chef at Launceston Place, a restaurant in London that was regularly haunted by politicians, English nobility and, most notably, by Princess Diana. In those days – and how dated this seems now – they had a delicious double-baked goat cheese soufflé starter. It never came off the menu and had also become a regular feature in many other restaurants. The only variation allowed was the sweet seasonal condiment that came with it. This is my little tribute to them and to '90s food.

Serves 6–10, depending on the size of
 your ramekins

Poached peaches

⅔ cup water

⅔ cup white wine

¾ cup sugar

½ tsp black peppercorns

½ vanilla pod, split and seeds scraped
 out

2 to 3 medium peaches, peeled

5 tbsp unsalted butter at room
 temperature, plus extra to brush
 the ramekins

½ cup ground hazelnuts

1 cup plus 2 tbsp milk

1 bay leaf

½ onion, studded with a few cloves

⅓ cup all-purpose flour

6 oz hard goat cheese (skin removed),
 broken into pieces

5 eggs, separated, plus 1 egg white

⅓ tsp salt

3 tbsp heavy cream per soufflé, if
 reheating

To make the poached peaches. Put all the ingredients in a medium saucepan (the peaches may not be totally covered with liquid; this is fine). Bring to a simmer and cook gently, covered, for about 15 minutes, turning the peaches over once. They need to be soft but shouldn't disintegrate. Leave them to cool down in the juices.

Preheat the oven to 375°F. Put a large roasting pan inside and pour into it enough boiling water to come ¾ inch up its sides. Take individual ramekins and brush their sides and bottoms with soft butter. Spoon in ground hazelnuts and turn the ramekins to coat the inside evenly. Remove any excess nuts and place the ramekins in the fridge.

In a small saucepan combine the milk, bay leaf and onion. Bring to the boil, then set aside. Take a medium saucepan, set on medium heat and melt the butter. Add the flour as you stir with a wooden spoon and cook while stirring for 2 minutes. Discard the bay leaf and onion and gradually add the milk to the butter mix as you stir. Continue cooking and stirring for 3 minutes as the mixture thickens. Off the heat, stir in the cheese, then the yolks and salt. Transfer to a mixing bowl.

In a separate bowl whisk the egg whites to soft peaks, then gently fold them into the cheese mix. Divide among the ramekins, filling them almost to the brim. Set them carefully in the pan of water in the oven. Bake for 10 to 12 minutes, or until golden brown and risen. You can now serve the soufflés directly from the oven.

Alternatively, turn off the oven and leave the soufflés inside for 10 minutes. Remove the pan from the oven and allow the soufflés to cool down in it. Now run a knife around the inside of the ramekins and take out the soufflés. Place, bottom side up, on a baking sheet lined with parchment paper (you can leave them there, covered, for up to 4 hours).

When ready to serve, preheat the oven to 325°F. Drizzle about 3 tablespoons of cream over each soufflé. Place the baking sheet in the oven and warm up well for about 8 minutes. Serve each soufflé with a few slices of peach (not too many!) drizzled with a little juice.

# Quince and sweet Gorgonzola salad

During a cooking class I gave at Leith's a few years ago a woman came up to me and said: "I've got a tree full of quinces in my garden but I don't do anything with them. I am scared of quince." She's not alone. The daunting thing about quince is the preparation. Although it has the innocent look of, say, an apple or a pear, it is rock hard and requires long cooking before becoming edible.

Still, once you've got rid of your quince aversion and tried preparing it yourself, you'll be amazed by the transformation it goes through, from an unyielding, dull, off-white, hard mass into a magnificent red fruit with a soft, perfumed flesh. You can then use it in plenty of contexts: in desserts or salads, or to accompany fatty and rich meats such as lamb, game or pork.

Any quince syrup left after making this salad (pictured on pages 276 to 277) you can warm up and pour over vanilla ice cream.

Serves 4 as a starter
1¾ cups water
1½ cups sugar
15 black peppercorns
4 strips of orange zest
2 bay leaves
juice of ½ lemon
¾ cup red wine
2 medium quinces
1 tsp grainy mustard
2 tsp cider vinegar
4 tbsp olive oil, plus extra to finish
salt and black pepper
2½ cups mixed leaves (such as mizuna, dandelion, watercress or radicchio di Treviso)
4 to 5 oz sweet Gorgonzola
scant ½ cup shelled unsalted pistachios, lightly toasted, some whole and some roughly chopped

Preheat the oven to 275°F. Take a medium-sized heavy pan that can go in the oven and for which you have a tight-fitting lid. Place inside the water, sugar, peppercorns, orange zest, bay leaves, lemon juice and red wine. Set on the stove and bring to a light simmer. As soon as the sugar dissolves, remove from the heat.

Meanwhile, use a vegetable peeler to peel the quinces; keep the skin. With a heavy knife, cut the fruit vertically into quarters and remove the core; keep this too. Cut each quarter into two segments. Place the quince segments, plus the skins and cores, in the sugar syrup. Cover the pan and put it into the oven to cook for about 2 hours. After this time the quince should be completely tender. Remove from the oven and leave to cool, uncovered.

Whisk together until smooth the mustard, vinegar, oil, 4 tablespoons of the quince cooking liquid, ½ teaspoon salt and a good grind of black pepper.

To finish the salad, place some salad leaves on four serving plates. Arrange four quince segments per portion and some hand-broken pieces of Gorgonzola on the leaves. Try to build the salad up. Place a few more leaves on top. Spoon the dressing over and scatter over the pistachios. Finish with a light drizzle of olive oil. Alternatively, arrange similarly in a large, central mixing bowl and bring to the table.

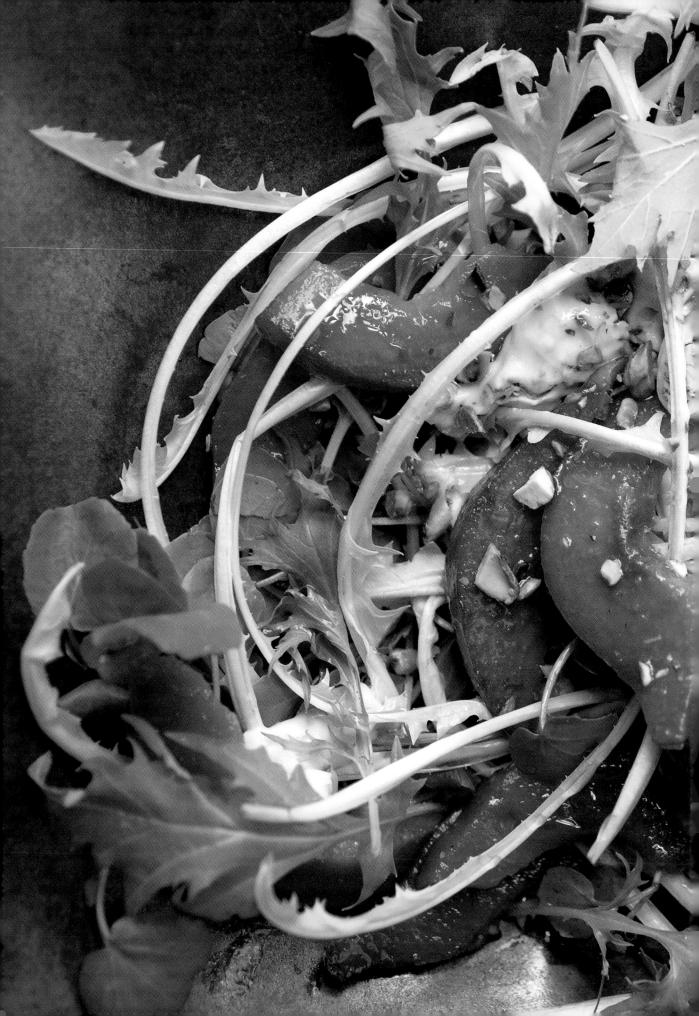

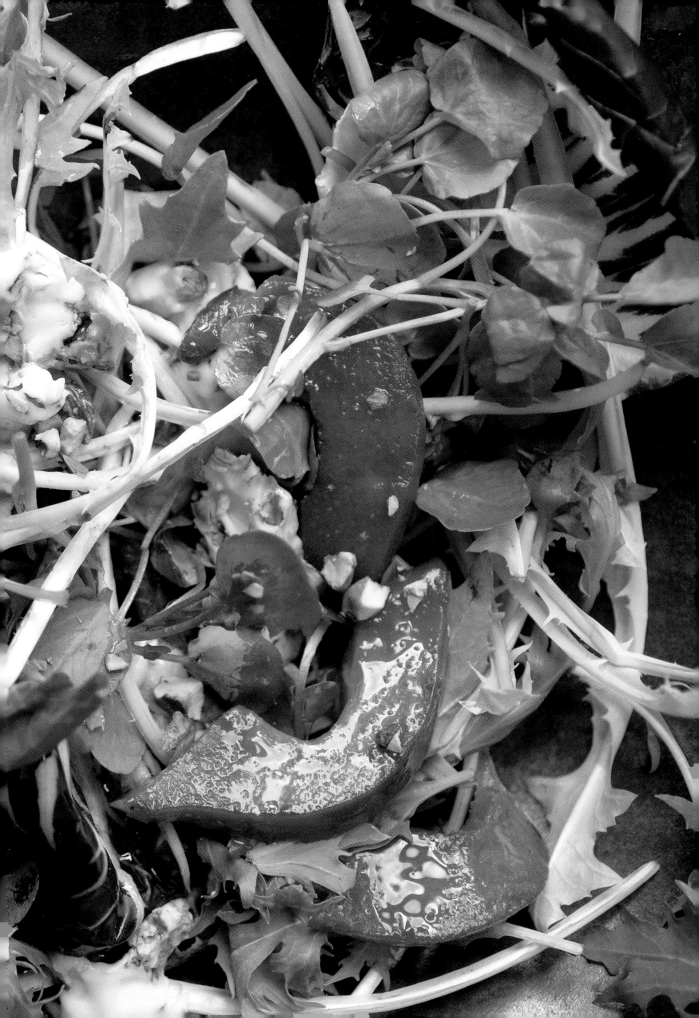

# Pear crostini

My dad always quotes an old Tuscan saying that was often used in conversation between a landowner and the supervisor of the land: *Al contadino non far sapere quanto è buono il formaggio con le pere*. The beautiful Italian melody unfortunately doesn't carry through to the English translation: To the peasant dare not tell how pears with cheese taste so well.

As well as revealing something about the class structure in the Italian countryside and about the existential anxieties of the landowners, the phrase also makes a much less explosive, but still profound, truth about the sublime combination of pear and cheese, particularly the Grandes Dames of Italian cheese, Parmesan and pecorino.

Here I go for goat cheese, which is just as good with pear when chosen well. It should be an artisanal one and full of flavor. You also need pears that are firm, yet sweet and slightly tart. Super-ripe pears, as much as I love them, will overcook and turn mushy.

Serves 4 generously
¼ cup pine nuts
5 tbsp olive oil, plus extra to finish
1 garlic clove, peeled
salt and black pepper
4 large slices sourdough bread, cut
    1½ inches thick
3 semi-ripe pears (unpeeled)
2 tsp sugar
2 tsp lemon juice
4 to 5 oz good-quality goat cheese
picked chervil leaves to garnish

Preheat the oven to 400°F. Place the pine nuts, 4 tablespoons of the olive oil, the garlic, a pinch of salt and some black pepper in the bowl of a food processor and work to a coarse and wet paste. Use a brush to apply to one side of every sourdough slice. Lay the bread slices on a baking sheet and bake for 10 minutes, or until lightly colored. Remove and allow to cool slightly.

While the bread is in the oven, prepare the pears. Stand each pear on a chopping board and use a sharp knife to trim off a very thin layer of the skin from each side. Then cut each pear lengthways into four thick slices. Remove the core with the tip of a knife. Place the slices in a bowl with the remaining 1 tablespoon of oil, the sugar, lemon juice and a pinch of salt. Toss gently.

Take a ridged griddle pan and place on a high heat until piping hot. Lay the pear slices gently in the pan and leave for about a minute on each side, just to make char marks. Turn carefully and then remove with tongs, trying not to break the pears.

To assemble the crostini, slice the cheese thinly and arrange over the toasts, alongside the pears. You want to be able to see both clearly, so allow them to overlap and rest on each other to create height. Place the crostini in the oven for 3 to 4 minutes, just to warm up and for the cheese to partly melt. Remove from the oven.

Garnish the crostini with the picked chervil leaves, drizzle with oil and sprinkle with freshly ground black pepper. Serve hot or warm.

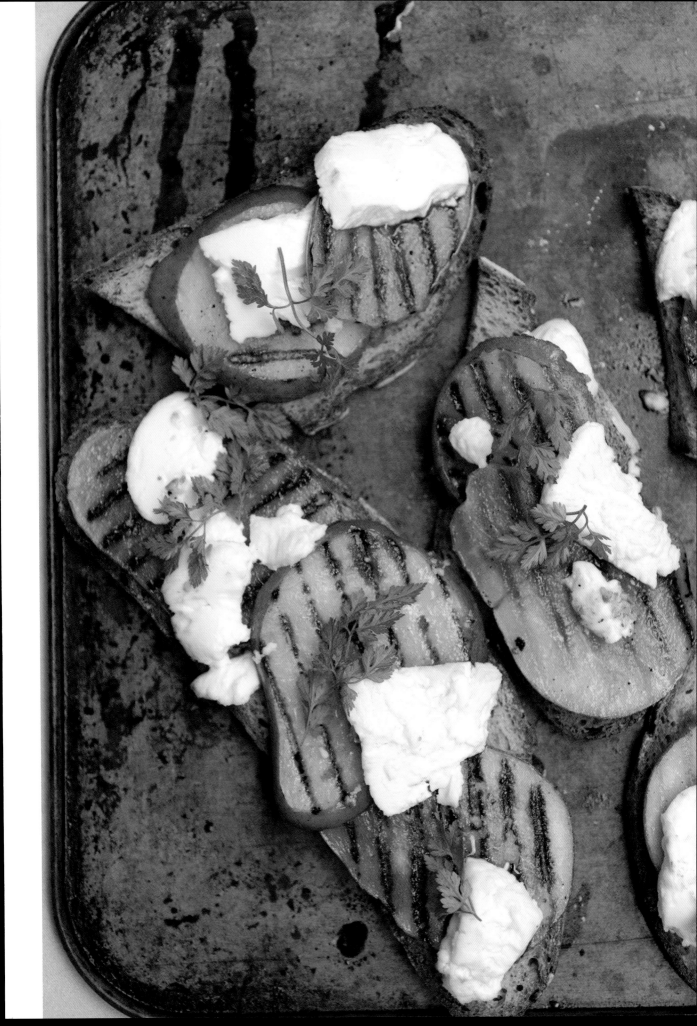

# Dates and Turkish sheep's cheese

Turkish grocers and supermarkets – there are many of them dotted around East and Northeast London – offer a bountiful selection of fresh and flavorful produce that you can never find in a normal supermarket. The vegetables are usually bursting with flavor, and you can also get some fantastic fresh breads and many dried products from all over the Balkans.

I go to the Turkish Food Center in Dalston, near Ottolenghi in Islington, for their wonderful cheeses. There are, literally, dozens of varieties on offer – mostly white young cheeses in brine. They are available from the cheese counter, where they float in wonderfully murky waters that keep them fresh and moist, but also in jars, plastic wraps, vacuum-packed and even cans. Think feta, halloumi or ricotta and then extend the range of flavors and textures tenfold. Some are creamy and light, others salty and crumbly. Some you can slice and fry, others spread like cream cheese. The best, I find, are the sheep's milk cheeses. Ask to taste from the counter or just gamble with the pre-packed varieties. You can't go far wrong.

Serves 4 as a starter
1½ tbsp whole almonds (skin on)
6 large Medjool dates (5 oz in total)
2½ cups arugula
4 to 5 oz lightly salted Turkish sheep's cheese (or buffalo ricotta or buffalo mozzarella), broken or cut into pieces
a few leaves of dill
¾ cup mixed purple and green basil leaves, and red chard leaves
3 tbsp olive oil
1½ tsp pomegranate molasses
salt and black pepper

Preheat the oven to 300°F. Spread the almonds in a small baking pan and roast them for 8 to 10 minutes, or until they turn a nice brown inside. Remove from the oven and leave to cool down.

Halve the dates lengthways and remove and discard the pit. Cut each half into four to six long slices.

Spread the arugula over the bottom of each serving dish. On top, build up dates, cheese, dill, basil and red chard, making sure you can clearly see all four elements.

Mix together well the olive oil, pomegranate molasses and some salt and pepper, and drizzle over the salad. Roughly chop the almonds, sprinkle on top and serve.

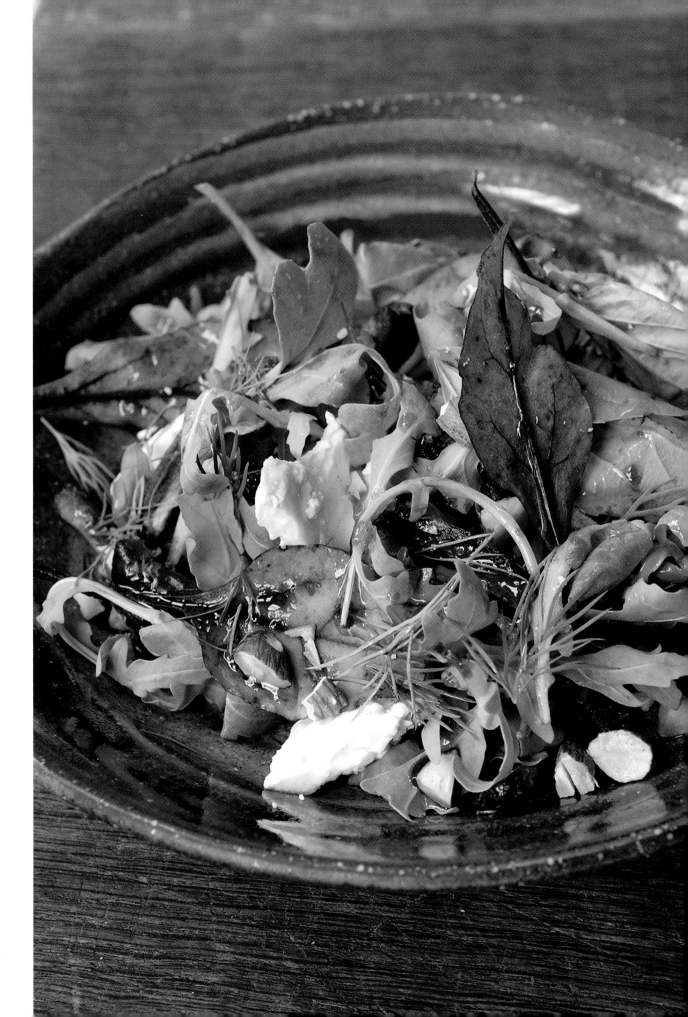

# Watermelon and feta

This you must eat on the beach, or at least outdoors, on a hot day, with the sun's rays unobstructed. It reminds me of hot sweaty nights on the seafront in Tel Aviv, when everyone is out enjoying beer, loud music and often a heated conversation. The sweet juiciness of the watermelon and the crumbly saltiness of the feta give this salad all its character. So make sure you choose the best possible of both (for other salty cheeses you can use here, see Dates and Turkish Sheep's Cheese, page 280).

Serves 4
10 oz feta
4½ cups large chunks of watermelon
¾ cup basil leaves
½ small red onion, very thinly sliced (optional)
olive oil

Slice the feta into large but thin pieces, or just break it by hand into rough chunks.

Arrange all the ingredients, except the olive oil, on a platter, mixing them up a little. Drizzle over some oil and serve at once.

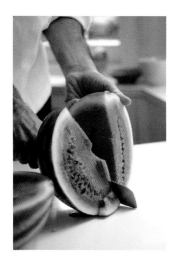 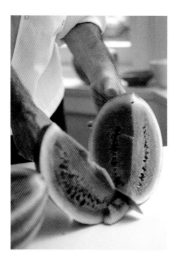

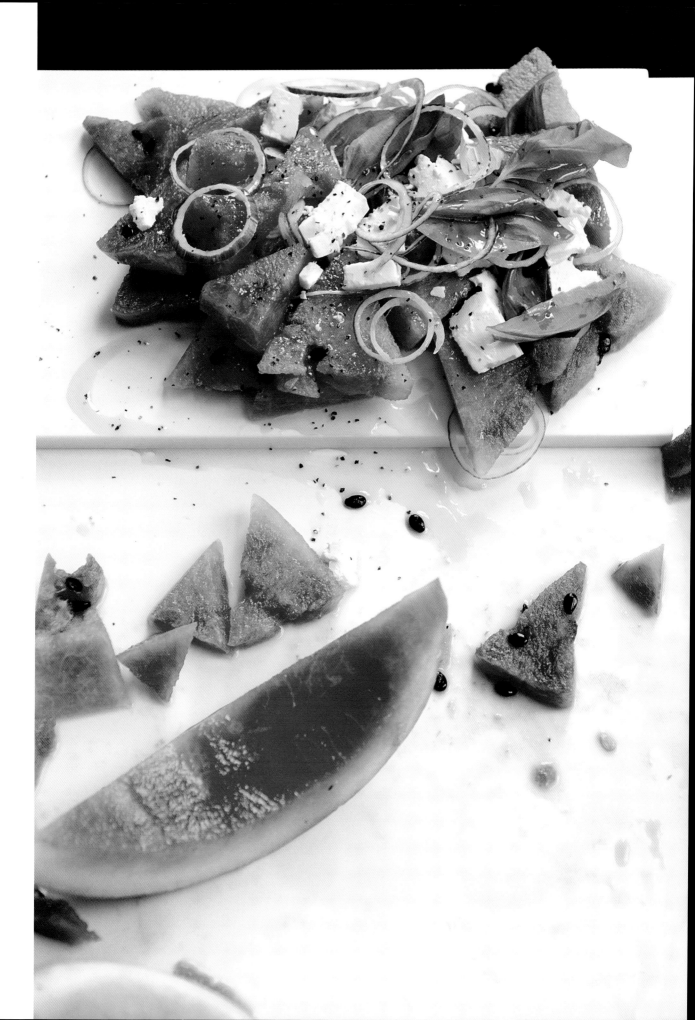

# Index

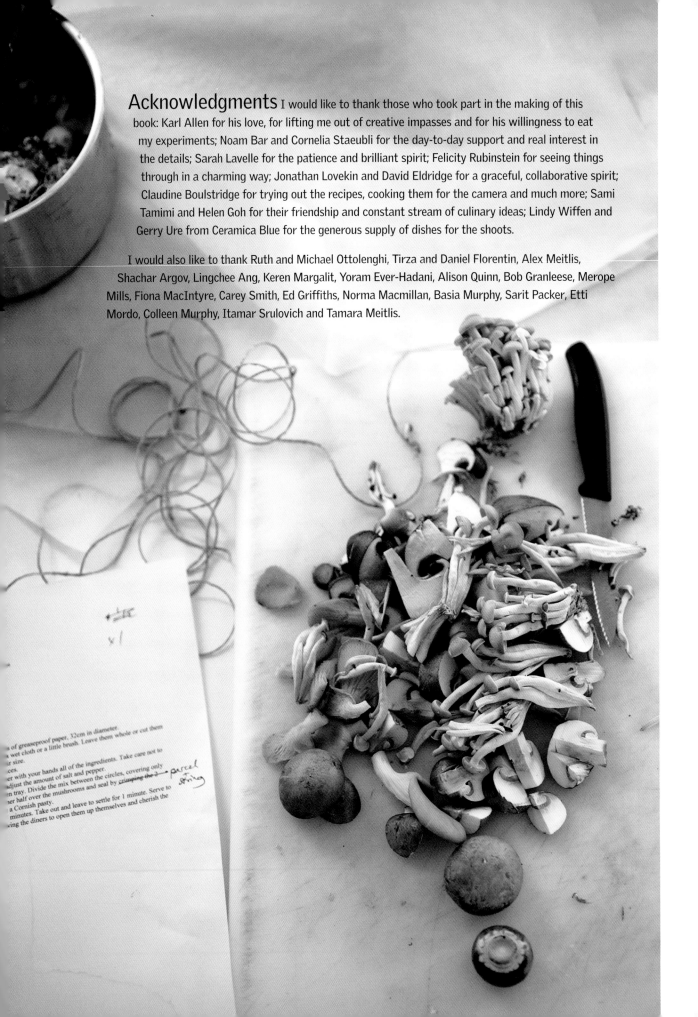

## Acknowledgments

I would like to thank those who took part in the making of this book: Karl Allen for his love, for lifting me out of creative impasses and for his willingness to eat my experiments; Noam Bar and Cornelia Staeubli for the day-to-day support and real interest in the details; Sarah Lavelle for the patience and brilliant spirit; Felicity Rubinstein for seeing things through in a charming way; Jonathan Lovekin and David Eldridge for a graceful, collaborative spirit; Claudine Boulstridge for trying out the recipes, cooking them for the camera and much more; Sami Tamimi and Helen Goh for their friendship and constant stream of culinary ideas; Lindy Wiffen and Gerry Ure from Ceramica Blue for the generous supply of dishes for the shoots.

I would also like to thank Ruth and Michael Ottolenghi, Tirza and Daniel Florentin, Alex Meitlis, Shachar Argov, Lingchee Ang, Keren Margalit, Yoram Ever-Hadani, Alison Quinn, Bob Granleese, Merope Mills, Fiona MacIntyre, Carey Smith, Ed Griffiths, Norma Macmillan, Basia Murphy, Sarit Packer, Etti Mordo, Colleen Murphy, Itamar Srulovich and Tamara Meitlis.

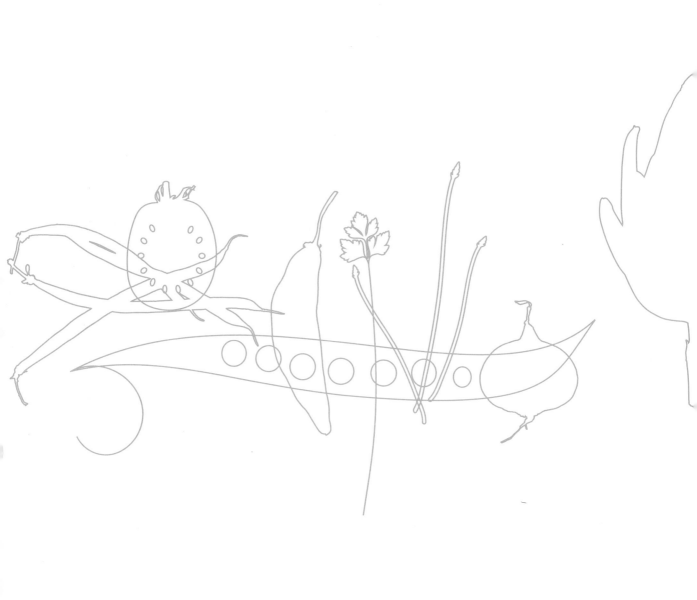